Copyright © 2024 by Dave Blackwell

All rights reserved.

Cover and Book design by Dave Blackwell

No part of this book may be reproduced in any form or by any electronic or mechanical means including information storage and retrieval systems, without permission in writing from the author. The only exception is by a reviewer, who may quote short excerpts in a review.

This book is a work of non-fiction. Names, characters, places, and incidents either are products of the author's experiences. No names or details of any persons have been mentioned or shared, only my own.

Dave Blackwell

Contact: dave.blackwell@live.co.uk

Printed Globally.

First Printing: February 2024

The Frustrations of Being Deaf

Part Two

A little about me...

If you have read part one – then you will know what you are getting yourself into. If not, then here is a brief outline again – but I recommend you check out part one!

I decided to put together this book of true stories, after experiencing so many funny, frustrating, and awkward moments (most of my deaf life!) however the pandemic made things worse. I work for the NHS as a Medical Engineering Specialist. Being deaf, I rely on lipreading and my implant to go about my normal day, however, life is currently far from normal...

Born in Dartford, England in 1977. I went deaf at the age of seven, my left side overnight and the right side over several months.

In 2011, I was in Florida and left my hearing aid out due to a nasty ear infection, a few days later I couldn't hear anything and put it down to a faulty hearing aid. Three months later after trying to get an urgent(!) appointment with my audiologist, it was discovered that I lost all hearing on my left side. Having not been given any options, I had to fight to see a specialist, eventually being referred to London for a Cochlear implant, which gave me back a huge percentage of hearing.

I hope you enjoy this book. Reading about the crazy people I meet, the situations I find myself in and most of all, the way I deal with them.

Being blunt, and treating everything as a joke... (Well nearly everything!) (Okay, mostly everything!) Enjoy this second batch of even more craziness!

1984 – LOSING MY HEARING

Dave is seven years old and stands at the sink, wearing nothing but boxers. He held his head to the side under the sink, the icy water running into my right ear. His face screwed up in fear, frantically crying. Turning off the tap he stepped away from the sink and sat down on the floor, his back against the bath. He buried his head in his knees and sobbed.

"Dave!" The woman yelled from a distance. Dave didn't respond. "Dave hurry up, you are going to miss the minibus!" The woman yelled again, louder and angrier.

Dave looked up and rested his head against the bath, breathing against sobs. His face is red and tears well in his eyes.

Dave stared at the door, shocked and lost. A tear ran down his face. After a few moments, he stood up. Looking in the mirror. He opened and closed his jaw as if he were trying to chew something large at the back of his mouth.

"One two three…." He said quietly to himself. He put his hand up to his left ear and covered it.

"One two three…." He said again, frustration on his face. He grunted in anger and fear as he started to hit himself in the ear. He sniffed, washed his face, and left the bathroom.

Dave looked out of the window of the minibus; the rain was coming down heavily. He watched the traffic. His eyes red from crying, he sniffed and sat back in the chair. He was hungry and tired. He hadn't had breakfast.

His throat was raw from crying. His head hurt, piercing headaches. His ears were full of noises.

Bells, whistles, buzzes.

He cupped his right ear and whined.

He could hear what was like voices in his head. A mixture of voices. Random and overlapping. He breathed harder, trying to make the noises go away. He moaned in frustration.

"You ok Dave?" A man's concerned voice.

Dave didn't respond. Still looking out the window and quietly crying to himself. His hand cupped over his right ear as he tried to hide from the world.

"Dave?" The voice again, this time the man placed his hand on Dave's shoulder.

Dave jumped in fright and wiped his eyes. He looked at the man who sat down in the vacant seat next to him.

The man was no older than forty, wearing a brown suit, and a cream shirt that was open at the collar. He had a well-groomed beard.

He smiled at Dave and Dave tried to smile back, but his bottom lip quivered as he tried not to cry. Dave hated people seeing him cry, he always hid it or forced himself not to cry.

"What's up, mate?" The man asked.

Dave looked at him, confused and lost. The man's voice was muffled. Dave couldn't hear anything out of his right ear, and his left ear was as if it were half-blocked. He could see the man speak but couldn't make out what he was saying.

The man looked at Dave, concerned and confused.

"Dave?" He said.

Dave burst into tears and looked away. He stared out of the window, Crying. Tears streamed down his face.

"What's wrong mate?" The man looked around, the other children becoming aware. Dave's sobbing filled the quietness of the bus.

Dave never got to class that day. He was taken to sickbay at the school by the coach driver who was concerned about what had happened. The school nurse arrived moments later to find Dave sitting on a chair in the corner of the sickbay, crying. His knees pulled up to his chest.

Nurse Janet was a short, athletic-built woman who had just celebrated her thirtieth birthday. She had arrived late to work due to oversleeping, one too many glasses of wine the night before most likely. She removed her bright red raincoat and hung it over a chair. Grabbing some tissues, she walked over to Dave and bent down in front of him, facing him. She was wearing black trousers and a light blue blouse. Her ginger curly hair was wet, and water ran down her face.

"Morning Dave." She smiled. "Take these and wipe your face. Let me dry up a little and I will be with you straight away." She spoke slowly and clearly. Dave took the tissues and nodded. Janet left the room and moments later came back with a white hospital towel, drying her hair. Draping it over the chair on her coat, she grabbed a stool next to the table and walked over to Dave, she placed it down and sat on it. Looking at Dave and smiling at him.

"So. What is wrong with you today?" Janet asked, unsure what the problem was. She arrived at the reception area and was told there was a sick child in the sick bay. She didn't ask any questions; however, she complained about the student being left on his own.

Dave began to cry.

"Come on love no more tears. I promise if you tell me what's wrong, you will begin to feel better. I promise." Janet said smiling.

"I cannot hear," Dave explained, pointing to his ears.

"Oh dear, let's have a look, shall we?" Janet said and got up. She picked up an otoscope from her desk. Switching it on and checking the light against her hand. She then sat back down.

5

"Are you in any pain with your ears?" She asked.

Dave shook his head to say no and put his legs down. He began to feel more at ease.

"Can I have a quick look in your ears please?" Janet asked.

"Yes," Dave said, sitting forward slightly.

Janet had a look in both of Dave's ears and after a few moments turned off the otoscope and put it on the trolley next to her.

"Your ears are very red. I will get in touch with your mum and dad and get them to take you to your doctor okay?" Janet said, placing her hand on Dave's knees.

"They are at work, they won't be home," Dave explained.

"What about someone else?" Janet said. Dave thought for a few seconds and then nodded.

"Nan," Dave said.

"Your nan. Ok, do you know her number?" Janet asked and picked up a pad and pen. Dave nodded and took the pen, writing the number down whilst Janet held the pad.

"Can I have some water?" Dave asked, his throat dry and raw.

"Of course, you can silly. Help yourself." Janet said with a smile, pointing to the water cooler in the corner of the room. "I'll call Nan for you and explain everything," Janet said reassuringly.

This day still sticks in my mind, going to my grandmothers and waiting until my parents came home, and then going to the doctors who started the process of finding out I was going deaf.

MY right ear went overnight, that was the most traumatic part. My left ear lost hearing slowly over a month, during this time I had tests and eventually was diagnosed with severe hearing loss, the reasons unknown at the time.

I received generic hearing aids for both ears and offered to take up sign language, but my parents declined. I met with a speech therapist to start learning how to lipread, however had already picked this up.

I didn't get the support I should have, especially from my local hospital or audiology, this contributed to issues with confidence and my learning, I struggled at school for years until a stranger stepped in to change things and get me the help I needed.

ALARMS

Security alarm

I always struggle with unknown noises and where they are coming from, for as long as I can remember.

I stayed late at work to catch up on some odds and ends, enjoying the peace after everyone else had gone home. Listening to music in the background, closing reports, and sending some emails.

I went to the kitchen and made myself a coffee, wondering what the quiet beeping sound was, trying to listen and focus on it with no luck. I checked the cupboard, the fridge, and even the urn, but couldn't work out where it was coming from.

   "Bugger it," I said to myself.

I walked out into the warehouse, holding my coffee and listening, it was faint. I opened the shutter door, listening but the sound of lorries and cars drowned out quieter noises.

I gave up and returned to my desk, spending half an hour, or so finishing up.

I decided to use the toilet before I left, learning my lesson after getting stuck on the duel carriageway and bursting for the loo.

And that is when I realized.

The building alarm had somehow turned itself on and was now going off, probably due to me setting it off earlier. No idea how long it had been going off, or even how it came to turn on. I reset it, trying to work out what the hell had happened. I checked with a colleague to find out if they had accidentally set it, but they hadn't.

Unsure why, but most likely it had been an on-auto set at a certain time of the day, I haven't stayed that late since, but at least I know now. The other issue is, why didn't anyone turn up with the alarms blasting?

Servicing

Another incident was when I got in early on a site to get their equipment serviced before the lists started. I get up at silly o'clock every day, which allows me to get things done or get some writing in, (like I am doing now).

I went up to the endoscopy ward, realizing the door was locked and I barely remembered the code. Lucky for me, a joke with one of the staff reminded me, that it was the year of her birth.
I put the code in and managed to get in.

Firstly there was an alarm blaring and I had never heard it before. I then checked the fire alarm panel, which was clear, so I had no idea what it was.

"I cannot work with that noise," I said to myself. "Might as well fix the light source first."

I went into the treatment room and removed the light source module so I could replace the lamp, something that would be easier to do in the workshop.

On the way to the workshop, I popped into security to let them know, but no one was in. So I went and replaced the lamp, having a coffee before returning.

As I left the workshop, a receptionist from the department and a security officer joined me on the way as we got into the lift.

"Good morning," She said.
"Hi," I replied and nodded to the security.
"Where are you going?" She asked.
"Endoscopy," I said. "Need to do some repairs."
"We are headed up there now," She said. "I just came down to get security because the alarms are going off."
"Some idiot set them off," Security said.
"That would be me," I replied. "I had no idea there were security alarms."
"Oh no," The woman said. "We forgot to tell you."

"Sorry about that," I said. "I did pop to security but there was no one there."

"I was in the loo," the security guard said. "Gut rot."

"Lovely," I said. "I always get there early so I can start," I said to the receptionist. "Had no idea they had an alarm otherwise I would have waited."

"We had to start using it," She said. "One of the girls was on her own at the weekend and a patient from mental health got on, scared the living daylights out of her."

"Not good," I said. "Anyhow I am sorry."

The lift arrived and I followed them both into the department where she reset the alarm and the security officer looked at me like I had committed the crime of the century.

It was a funny conversation when I spoke to the nurse later, only to be told about a plonker setting off the alarms and scaring the receptionist.

I was that plonker, but at least I now know.

Alarms in the dark

It was around five in the morning and I was sitting on the mezzanine floor at work, writing. (For clarification, this was The Night Porter, a comedy, so do check it out.)

I had managed a thousand words, sipping at my coffee when a loud piercing alarm broke the silence, causing me to jump, and spill coffee onto my lap. I got to my feet, looking around for the source of the alarm.

"Where is it coming from?!" I muttered.

I waited for a few minutes, hoping it would turn off but it didn't, and my ears were beginning to ring.

I thought it was the building alarm, so I ran across the mezzanine floor in the dark, forgetting there was a glass jug in the middle under a ceiling leak. It let out a crash as it went skidding across the floor and crashed into the steel trunking around the pipework. I couldn't see it and ignored it, making my way into the upstairs office towards the stairs, reaching out for the door as I put my weight against it, to find it locked.

I bounced off the door and fell back onto the floor, jolting and knocking the air out of myself. Groaning as I lay there for about a minute, the muffled alarm still going.

I got up and unlocked the door, running down the stairs and stopping at the bottom when I could no longer hear the alarm. I checked the fire alarm panel and the security panel, and both were normal.

"Where is it coming from?" I said in frustration.

I walked through the workshop, listening, and then into the warehouse where the alarm greeted me. I looked around in the darkness, wondering what the hell it was.

"Time for the hearing aids to come out," I said and ran up the stairs, stopping when I noticed a red light through a score of ventilators in storage. That is when I realized what the alarm was. The unit had a battery failure due to having not been plugged in for so long and went into a failure state.

I got hold of it, pulling it out and lifting it. Attempting and failing to silence it, I plugged it in, sighing in relief when it stopped.

I then got back to my writing, struggling due to the alarm-induced tinnitus, which always has a way of ruining my day.

Security Blinder

Another early morning I decided to sit in the car and write when one of the local buildings started alarming, so I took my hearing aids out and just focused.

About ten minutes later, a light beams into the car and blinds me and someone is banging on the window.

I put my hearing aids in, turned the ignition, and put down the window.

"You are blinding me," I said. "Can you turn that off!"

The person spoke to me and I had no idea what they were saying.

"I am deaf," I said. "I need to lip-read you."

The man turned off his headlight and I had to blink several times to focus.

"Do you work here?" He asked.

"Yes," I said.

"How long has the alarm been going off?" He asked.

"I don't know," I replied. "Ten minutes or so."

"Did you call anyone?" He asked.

"No," I said. "Who are you?"

"Security," He showed me his badge. "Just wondering why you are sitting in the carpark."

"I work in there," I pointed to the warehouse. "Just waiting on a colleague."

"Do you have identification?" He asked me.

"Yes," I said. "Why?"

"Can you prove you work here?" He said.

"Well," I said showing him my badge and shirt with the logo on. "Shouldn't you be checking on the building instead of harassing me?"

"You were acting suspicious," He said. "Not responding when I spoke to you."

"Deaf," I said. "I need to lip-read."

"Okay," He said. "I will pop back later and confirm you work here."

"Fine by me," I said. "Make sure you bring coffee and doughnuts."

I closed the window and he hovered for a minute before walking away, making his way towards the alarming building.

He never did return to confirm.

Nor did he bring coffee and doughnuts, I was very disappointed.

11

Monitor Alarm

Another perfect example of not being able to track down where sound is coming from, even when it is right under my nose.

I was working on a monitor, changing the touchscreen due to it failing. It had been a while since I did one, so I was taking my time, trying to remember where all the problem cables were.

As I removed the batteries, the unit began to beep, so I then pressed the button and unplugged it from the extension lead, and another alarm sounded.

"Bloody hell!" I muttered, pressing the button on the side of the monitor, groaning when nothing happened. "Stop beeping!"

I tried everything to stop the beeping but had no luck, so I gave up and took my implant out so I could concentrate on swapping the screen without the thing alarming in my ear.

Just as I had nearly finished, awkwardly trying to get the final lead which you need tiny flipping hands to do, someone tapped me on the shoulder, causing me to jump.

It was one of the porters, talking to me. Well trying to.

"What's up?" I said, putting my implant back in.
"Thought you were ignoring me!" He said. "What's with the beeping?" He asked.
"I cannot stop it," I said. "Once I put the batteries in, it will be fine."
"It's not that," He said. "It's that!" He pointed to an uninterruptable power supply on the table, and then it hit me.

I reached over and pressed the power button, and the alarm stopped.

"Been going off for ages," He said. "Then I remembered you are deaf, so it's probably you!"
"I thought it was the monitor!" I groaned. "Bloody thing has been plugged in for months doing nothing!"
"You plonker!" He said.
"Thanks," I said grinning. "You okay?"

12

"Yeah," He said. "Can I borrow you in a minute?"

"Depends on what for!" I said curiously.

"Just meet me outside in a few minutes!" He said.

"I'll finish this and pop out," I replied. "Can you stay in the area in case any more alarms go off?"

Noises like that drive me crazy, new sounds that I hadn't heard before suddenly come to the service to annoy me. For example, the week of my implant switch on, I was constantly learning new noises, even if they did annoy the hell out of me.

I sat at my desk, wondering what the hell this humming noise was, it was irritating me.

When a colleague came in, I asked him and he pointed out a refrigerator in a locked room, at the end of the workshop!

It has worked wonders for me, but at the same time, annoying, especially with high heels, people eating, and beeping and buzzing mobiles!

The Frustrations of Being Deaf – Part Two

WAITING ROOMS AND ANTI-VAXXERS

I had the COVID-19 vaccine due to working in a hospital and being around vulnerable people and I had no concerns or issues with having it.

I was sitting in an Accident and Emergency waiting room after an accident at home, resulting in an ice burn to my arm and something in my eye, irritating the hell out of me. The waiting room was empty, however I was told there was still a wait to see a consultant.

A woman walked in, spoke to reception, and then sat opposite me in the waiting room, holding her hand with a bloodied bandage.

"Good morning," She said.

"Morning," I smiled. "How are you?"

"Sore," She held up her hand. "Carving knife!"

"Owch," I said. "Hope it isn't too bad."

"Thanks," she cradled her hand. "What about you?"

"Compressed gas can blew up yesterday," I showed her the blister on my arm.

"Oh, that looks nasty!" She hissed.

"And I have something in my eye that is irritating me," I kept blinking.

"You work here," She noticed my top. "Don't you get fast-tracked?"

"No," I shook my head. "Wouldn't want to, to be honest."

"They said there is a waiting time," She shook her head. "Probably on breaks."

"It's a big place," I added. "A lot goes on behind the scenes that people don't see."

"Really," She said unimpressed. "What is that?" She asked curiously.

"What," I said looking outside behind me.

"That thing on your head," She pointed at the implant headpiece.

"Oh that," I chuckled. "It's my implant processor."

"Implant?" She said. "Is that like a pacemaker thing?"

"What?" I said. "On my head?"

"Well I don't know," She scoffed.

"It's a hearing aid," I said. "I am deaf."

"Shouldn't it be on your ear?" She scoffed and rolled her eyes.

"No," I said. "That is where the coil is. It is a cochlear implant, that transfers sound to electrical signals and then my brain does the rest."

She looked dumbfounded and disgusted.

A nurse came from the triage room and called the woman in.

"At last!" She said. "Bye!"

I sat back in the chair and closed my eye, it was irritating and sore, I just wanted it to stop so I could get back to work.

A few minutes later, the woman walks out of the triage room, unhappy and verbal about it.

"Shocking service here," She complained. "They said that I now have to wait to see someone else!"
"Quite normal," I said. "First they triage and then assign you to the relevant person."
"No wonder the NHS is a mess," She said sitting down opposite me. "How long does it take to pop in a couple of stitches so I can go home?" She groaned. "My poor daughter has to do her breakfast and her lunch herself!"
"Oh dear," I said trying to be sympathetic. "How old is she."
"Fifteen," She said. "Poor girl."
"I am sure she will be fine," I said, shocked that a poor fifteen-year-old would have to make their lunch, what is the world coming to? (Sarcasm obviously)
"She cannot even cut bread!" The woman exclaimed. "That is how I got this!" She held up her hand again. "Cutting bread."
"With a carving knife?" I said curiously.
"Yes," She nodded. "The bread knife was in the dishwasher."
"Okay," I bit my tongue.
"They also asked if I had the poison jab!" She scoffed.
"Poison jab?" I said. "What is that?"
"The vaccine!" She said. "For this flu thing."
"Oh you mean the COVID-19 vaccine?" I said. "Fair enough."
"You better not have it," She said. "You might lose your hearing that you have left!" She gasped. "Or get more disabled!"
"I can't lose any hearing," I replied. "I am completely deaf."

15

"No you are not," She shook her head.

"I am," I said. "Trust me I know my own hearing issues."

"But you can hear me!" She exclaimed. "Surely you cannot fake that."

"Cochlear implant," I said. "That gives me my hearing."

"Well the jab will probably cancel it out," She warned me.

"Don't be silly," I said. "I already had it."

She groaned and shook her head.

"So what else is wrong with you?" She asked.

"Nothing," I said.

"I heard that some men are sterile, and some cannot even get it up, can you?" She demanded.

"I am not sharing that with you," I said.

"Worried I am right?" She asked.

"No," I said. "I'd consider educating yourself before you spew rubbish in public though."

"Rude," She said. "I might complain about you."

"I don't care," I got up and sat at the opposite end of the waiting room, secretly hoping they would stitch up her mouth.

Half an hour later, I was called in by a consultant. It was not a straightforward session, she couldn't examine my eyes with the slit lamp due to it being out of order, after putting the drops in my eye, she then disappeared and I thought I had been forgotten about. Fifteen minutes later she came back, stating she had been called away, and forgot about me. A nurse came in with four ophthalmoscopes, dragging the heads and complaining they were faulty and had been reported (They hadn't).

After all that, they had to do the drops again. They confirmed there was nothing in my eye, however it was still irritating me. She said to come back in an hour if it was still bad. So I left, no better off than when I came in.

An hour later I came back, my eye throbbing along with the huge blister on my forearm. The woman from earlier was still in the waiting room, sipping from a coffee and looking extremely bored.

After explaining things to a very unfriendly triage nurse, one of the consultants recognized me and called me in. I explained it to him and he pulled up my record, asking if I had used the drops.

Long story short, the original consultant had forgotten to prescribe me drops. So the consult did that, and also some cream for my arm.

The drops worked wonders.

The vax took my hearing

I met up with friends and gained the interest of someone, who seemed to want to know anything about my hearing disability.

"Hi," He said. "Not seen you around before."
"Lucky you," I laughed.
"What is that?" He pointed to my implant.
"A processor," I said. "I am profoundly deaf."
"Profoundly?" He asked curiously.
"Completely deaf," I said. "Without it, I cannot hear anything at all."
"Nothing?" He asked.
"No," I said.

He then did something, which tons of people have done and I always know what they have said. He covered his mouth and said....

"Can you hear what I am saying?" He said.
"Obviously," I said. "It has been done thousands of times and gets more boring every time."
"Touche," he said. "So you lip-read?" He asked. "What about signs?"
"I lip-read yes," I nodded. "Signs? The film or the ones outside on the road?"
"Funny!" He snorted. "The hand sign stuff?"
"Sign language," I said. "No, never learnt."
"How did you go deaf?" He asked.
"Unknown," I said. "But a geneticist states it was most likely dodgy genetics."
"Rubbish," He said. "Sounds like a cover-up."
"Cover up?" I said curiously.
"Bet it was the vaccine," He scoffed.
"The what?" I asked.

"The vaccine," He said. "So many people have been injured or killed by it."

"No," I said. "It had nothing to do with the vaccine."

"How do you know?" He asked. "Have you had it?"

"Yes," I nodded. "I had the vaccine and have had no issues."

"How do you know?" He demanded.

"Because I do," I said, trying to get away.

I walked to the bar to order a drink, and he was back along with his girlfriend.

"Is it true?" She asked.

"Is what true?" I said curiously.

"That your hearing loss is a vaccine injury," She said. "The covid vaccine."

"No," I said. "I went deaf in eighty-four."

They looked at each other and then back at me.

"Must have been another vax you had," She said.

"It was genetics," I said. "Let's change the subject."

"Genetics," She laughed.

I nodded.

"Both my parents had a dodgy hearing gene," I said. "I got both dodgy halves."

"Really?" He said looking at me. "How do you know?"

"A qualified geneticist," I said.

"We are not having the vaccine," She said. "It's a government thing."

"I'd recommend not breeding either," I said. "Never a good thing."

I avoided them for the rest of the night, they were absolutely nuts.

BUSES

The buses were running late as usual and when one finally turned up, it was full to the point that when I got on, I was standing next to the door.

A few minutes into the journey, a toddler's cries and screams echoed through the bus and I wished I didn't have my hearing aids in.

The bus stopped and the door opened, clipping the side of my shoulder. The driver looked at me, apologizing and speaking clearly, trying to sign, that he must have guessed I was deaf.

"It's okay," I said. "Hardly felt it."
"It's busy," He said. "So many people."

The kids' howls echoed through the bus.

A woman standing next to me shook her head.

"You are so lucky," She said.
"Why is that?" I asked.
"You cannot hear that," she rolled her eyes.
"I can," I said. "My hearing aids pick up everything!"
"I wish he would shut up," She said. "Maybe the driver should ask her to get off the bus."
"That is a bit extreme," I said. "Kids do that."

The driver looked at me, shaking his head.

"How deaf are you?" She asked, looking at the implant.
"Completely," I replied. "This gives me about eighty-five percent."
"Must be good to switch off?" She said.
"It is," I smiled.
"Why don't you have them on now?" she asked.
"Easier to have them on when in public," I said. "The general public is hard work when it comes to my hearing loss."

The rest of the journey was long and loud, and when I got into town I made my way to the bus stop to get my second bus, only for the woman with the toddler to be right behind me, my implant battery was certainly working hard that day.

I turned off my implant due to the combined noise of the traffic, people, and an extremely vocal toddler, I didn't fancy a headache for the evening. And I stood watching the monitor, the ten-minute countdown for my bus.

A few minutes passed and this random woman got in my face, angry and yelling.

I stepped back and turned my implant on.

>"Problem?" I asked.
>"Can I sit down?!" She said angrily.
>"Sure," I said, unsure why she was asking.
>"Then move!" She snapped. "Bloody rude!"
>"I didn't hear you," I replied.
>"I was right next to you!" She said.
>"I know," I stepped back again. "Right in my face. I am deaf."
>"Sure you are," She said and sat down.
>"Whatever," I scoffed, ignoring her.

She kept throwing comments at me, and people started to look around.

>"Can anyone else hear that irritating whining noise?" I asked. "Reall piercing isn't it."

The woman got up and walked away, randomly muttering and moaning.

>"Don't think she was all there mate," An older man in front of me said.
>"I think you are probably right," I replied. "Always get the crazies out and about."
>"I did tell her you were probably deaf," He said. "but she wouldn't have it."
>"No skin of my nose," I replied. "Some people tend to react badly when they realize, rather than let it go over their head."

I was home within half an hour and the hearing aids came off, silence for the rest of the evening.

A long day

One of my pet hate with buses is that they are either not on time, or they never show. One of the services I use, boasts of a bus every ten minutes, however on this day, I had been waiting for fifty minutes until two came along. One didn't stop, however, the one behind did, only it was full, so I ended up standing at the front.

On the second stop, I didn't realize how close I was to the doors and when they opened, they cracked the side of my head and sent my implant flying to the floor. Naturally, the idiots on the bus continued to get off, narrowly avoiding treading on it.

"Sorry mate," The bus driver said. "I am so sorry."
"It's fine," I said. "My fault."
"Is it broken?" He asked.
"No," I checked it. "It's all good."

The driver was clearly spoken, so I wondered if he knew deaf people or had some experience.

A few stops later when all the feral kids got off, a few seats became available, so I sat down. I removed my implant and put it away and proceeded to play a game on my phone.

Ten minutes or so passed, and considering it was cold, I suddenly felt a warm blow on my right ear.

I had a fright when I turned around, to find a man standing inches away from my face, yelling.

I put my implant back in, expecting him to ask if he could sit next to me.

"Yes?" I said.
"Why are you ignoring me?" He demanded. "So rude!"
"I wasn't," I replied.
"You were!" He shouted. "Everyone can see you were!"
"I am deaf," I said to him and before I could speak further, he started yelling.

"I don't care, that is no reason to ignore someone!" He yelled.

"You do realize that deafness is unintentional ignorance?" I said.

A few people laughed.

"Don't get smart with me!" He grunted. "Not in the mood!"

"What did you want?" I asked.

"I want to sit there," He said.

"But there are two empty seats over there," I pointed to the two sets of two seats, both empty. "And I am sitting here."

"Can you move or what?" He snapped.

"Or what," I said.

"I am going to complain," He snapped, walking away.

I watched as he went to the bus driver and complained, and after a few heavy words, he walked off the bus, punching the window next to me as he walked past.

"Must have been Wayne," I said. "Bit of an odd one."

"I did say you may have been deaf," an old woman behind me said. "He just proceeded to shout."

At the next bus stop, a woman got on with a buggy and two children. As soon as she saw the two people sitting at the front, she proceeded to scream at them.

"I need that spot," She shouted. "I have a buggy, move!" She screamed.

The two people looked up in confusion, considering the spot opposite them was free.

"I said move," She yelled. "I am a mother with a buggy, are you blind or something?!"

"Looks like Wayne's other half, Waynetta!" I said, causing a few laughs.

"What was that?" She snapped.

"I am on my phone," I replied. "Could you keep it down thanks."

"I am a mother!" She snapped. "People need to be more understanding."

"No comment," I muttered to myself, and at this point, the implant came out.

22

I had the unfortunate encounter of getting off at the same bus stop, and then trying to get past her as she pushed the buggy, dragged the kids, and faffed on her phone.

The wildlife on buses is crazy, plenty of writing material there.

CAGE VS ME

I was in a supermarket, grabbing a few things midweek for lunch due to the fact I had left mine on the worktop in a hurry.

I grabbed a couple of pasta bowls, crisps and a drink and made my way to the self-service checkouts.

I suddenly realised I fancied some cheese, so I turned around and headed for the cold section. I found some Babybel cheese, only just!

I hurried back to the checkouts, walking past a cage when something suddenly caught me on the side of the head, knocking me off balance.

My implant suddenly lost power, and my hand went to my head due to the sharp pain.

I turned around when I realised my implant wasn't on my head, looking everywhere for it, before looking up at the girl holding a cage door, visibly upset.

"I am okay," I said. "I have lost my hearing aid," I said pointing to my ear.

I still had my basic hearing aid in my right ear, so I could hear a little enough to manage.

"I am very sorry," she said. "It was jammed and flipped open!" She said, nearly in tears.
"It's okay," I reassured her. "Can you look out for a hearing aid?"
"Is it the same as that one?" She asked, pointing to my right ear.
"No," I said. "It's an implant processor, black with a small cable and headpiece, the size of a two-pence coin."

We looked everywhere, under the cage, under the refrigeration units, and the length of the aisle in case someone had accidentally kicked it and sent it sliding, however, we couldn't locate it. She called for a supervisor to help out, and we searched high and low. Even some members of the public joined in the search.

"Is this part of it?" The girl came up to me and handed me a battery.

"Yes," I said. "Just the rest of it now!"

"Where was it?" The supervisor asked.

"A customer found it down the bottom," She pointed at the bottom of the aisle.

"I am sorry," She said. "I am stupid."

"It was an accident," I added. "It is insured."

The supervisor called a manager who wanted to record what had happened and take down my details, offering to compensate if needed.

I had given him all the information when something caught my eye.

At the bottom of the cage, I could see my implant processor swinging back and forth as a member of the team stacked cardboard.

"Hold on," I said and got down on my knees, popping the magnet off the cage.

"Is that it?" The supervisor said. "Nice spot!"

I plugged the battery in and connected it to my head, luckily enough, it worked fine.

"Is it okay?" the girl asked, her eyes red from the earlier tears.

"All good," I said. "Panic over."

"Do you want to take a complaint further?" The manager asked.

"No," I said. "Accidents happen, that cage has seen better days."

"I will run your things through free of charge," He said. "Least we can do."

"Thank you," I said.

I hugged the girl, it must have been a traumatic experience slamming a cage door against my head.

Was a little sore the next day, however, no harm was done.

I was more upset about my melted ice cream.....

CAR MOT

I always seem to have issues getting my yearly MOT with a garage, mainly because from experience, they all struggle with understanding what a hearing disability is.

This was my second year with this garage and I booked an appointment and turned up at the requested time.

The man behind the counter was not happy to see me, or a person in general, I have no idea.

> "Yes?" He said bluntly.
> "I have an appointment," I said, giving him my name and registration. "MOT and Service."
> "Okay," He nodded. "Key," He held out his hand.

I handed him the key.

> "How long will it be?" I said.
> "Come back tomorrow," He said.
> "I have a waiting appointment," I replied. "Same day."
> "We are busy," he said.
> "Not really my problem," I said. "I need the car tomorrow and I booked a slot."

The man sighed and walked into the workshop, returning a few minutes later.

> "Three hours," He said.
> "Could you text or email me when it's done?" I asked him.
> "No," He said. "We call you."
> "I cannot use the phone," I replied. "It has to be text or email."
> "What do you mean you cannot use the phone?" He looked at me. "It's simple."
> "I am deaf," I replied.
> "Then I can shout," He shrugged his shoulders. "Not a problem."
> "That doesn't help," I said.
> "Helps my mother," He said. "She is deaf."
> "I am not your mother," I said. "And it doesn't help."

"We cannot email you," He said.

"But you did the other day," I said. "So why is it a problem now."

At this point, another man came in behind the counter.

"Okay," he said. "I will text you."

"I will be back in three hours or so," I said and left.

I walked into town, twenty minutes away and sat in a coffee shop, watching videos on my phone. After a while I chilled out, watching the world go by and when I looked at my phone, I had three missed calls from an unknown number.

"I wonder," I said and googled it, finding it was the garage.

I then walked back to the garage, getting annoyed on the way. I had only been gone an hour, so unlikely they had finished it.

The man came behind the counter, looking at me and then looking down at the computer.

"You called me?" I said.

"Yes," He nodded.

"So you ignored everything I said when I spoke to you earlier?" I was annoyed.

"Well you came back," He seemed unbothered. "What is the issue."

"Is the car done?" I asked.

"No," He said. "We don't have the equipment to do it."

"So why did you accept the booking?" I asked. "This is annoying."

"Happens," He said. "You will have to rebook it."

"Can you give me a date?" I asked.

"No," He said. "You will need to call and book it."

"I think I need to contact head office and tell them about your attitude and discriminative behaviour," I said. "You have done nothing but give me grief and crappy service since I walked in."

"it's nothing personal," He said. "We cannot meet the needs of everyone."

"Definitely an official complaint," I said. "Going to have a fun time reporting this on social media later."

A mechanic came in from the workshop and I recognised him from the year before.

"What is going on?" He asked. "Problem?"

"Just this guy discriminating against me because I am deaf," I replied.

"No I didn't," the man said.

"I asked for texts or emails," I said. "Because I cannot hear on the telephone, you ignored this and called me three times."

"Did you?" He said.

"I am sure the camera will back me up," I pointed to the camera. "Key," I held out my hand.

"A please would be nice," The man said.

"I agree, something you could have tried earlier," I grinned. "This place will make a huge improvement if they get rid of the unprofessionalism."

"Go out the back," the mechanic said. "I will sort this out."

The mechanic was so much more professional, telling me that the man behind the counter was going through a bad time.

I booked the appointment, over email, a month later, that is how long I had to wait for them to deal with it because the garage forgot and called me a few times.

I made a complaint and they said they would 'Look at training their staff in recognising customer needs' which actually means, we will ignore it.

Time for a new garage.

CINEMA

It was a Friday evening after work, and I headed to the local shopping centre to grab some food and see a film.

The cinema was quite busy, and I got some snacks and water and made my way to my seat to get comfortable.

I hadn't slept the night before, so I was hoping I wouldn't nod off, I was already regretting seeing the film once I sat down and the tiredness hit me.

I managed to survive and halfway through the film, I noticed someone standing next to me and then shining a torch in my face, several people complained, looking at me as if I had done something wrong. I then followed the man outside, so I could properly understand him.

When I got into the foyer, I realised it was a security officer who had asked me to come outside, and by the counter were the police.

"Problem?" I asked.
"Is there a reason you were ignoring the staff?" The man asked me.
"What staff?" I asked.
"One of the team came in to confirm your seat, only for you to ignore her," The security officer said. "You were extremely rude."
"Okay," I said. "I didn't ignore anyone."
"So why didn't you respond?" He asked.
"Profoundly deaf in both ears," I said. "Implant on that side, nothing on the other side."

The security officer was lost for words, looking at the girl behind the counter.

"Did you call the police for me?" I asked.
"We thought you were going to be a problem," He said. "So you cannot hear anything?"
"Not in a cinema," I said.
"She said she had a torch on you and everything," He said.
"No," I replied. "That isn't true, if I had seen a torch, I would have noticed her standing there."

"Wait here," He said, making his way over to the counter.

One of the police officers made his way over to me.

"Everything okay sir?" He asked. "I hear there have been some issues?"
"No," I said. "Just lack of common sense."
"How do you mean?" He asked.
"Someone spoke to me in the cinema," I said. "I am deaf, so because I couldn't hear them, they have called the police and pulled me out of the film."

The officer looked at his colleague, shaking his head. The security officer then walked over, looking uncomfortable.

"Looks like we made a mistake," He said. "We apologise, you can go back inside."
"I would rather have a refund," I said. "I have already missed part of the film and you did a good job of making me look like a villain in there."
"We can arrange a refund," He said.

He led me over to the counter, along with the officer.

"Could you organise a refund for this gentleman please?" He said to the girl.
"I had no idea," she said. "I am sorry."
"That's fine," I replied. "Awareness has a long way to go."
"Do you not wear a badge or anything?" She said.
"A badge for what?" I asked.
"Well to let people know you are deaf?" She said.

The police officer chuckled, shaking his head.

"You want disabled people labelled?" I said. "Really?"
"I didn't mean it like that," She smiled awkwardly.
"What about prison camps?" I said. "Separate toilets?"
"Now you are being silly," She said.
"I think we may need a supervisor," The security officer said.

The girl walked away and after a minute a young man turned up.

"What do you need?" He asked.

"Could you refund this gentleman please," The security officer asked.

The police left at this point and I handed the ticket to the guy behind the counter.

"I cannot refund this," He said. "The film has already started."

"We pulled him out due to a misunderstanding," The officer said. "Refund him please."

"I will have to run this through with my manager first," He said.

"Or I can generate some amazing publicity about the discrimination that I have experienced," I said. "I am sure the local papers would enjoy it, along with all the social media accounts I have."

He looked at me and then at the security officer.

"My hands are tied," He said. "I cannot do anything."

"Okay," I shrugged my shoulders. "I will email the manager tomorrow and let him have a link to all the posts online."

"Hold on," The security guard said. "Can you do anything?"

"No," The man said.

"What is the point in making you a supervisor?" The security officer scoffed.

"You on Twitter?" I asked him.

"Yes," he said. "Why?"

"Check it out tonight when I tweet about the incompetent and discriminative staff," I said. "Deaf people not welcome at the so and so cinema!"

"Let me go and make a call," He said.

"You know what," I said in annoyance. "I am going to go," I said. "I am tired and fed up."

"I am sorry you feel that way," He said.

"Ticket please," I said.

"I have to retain this," He said.

"I paid for that," I said. "Or are you retaining the evidence to deny things?"

The security guard took the ticket and handed it to me.

"This place has gone downhill," I said. "Thanks for ruining my evening."

The next day I emailed the manager, who blamed the issues on technical problems. However after I said that there was no technology to blame, he then said he would update the staff training and awareness.

Turns out that the girl had read the incorrect seat number, and someone had said I was in the wrong seat, which I wasn't. I received a nice gift voucher for my trouble, not been back since.

COLD CALLERS

I never wear my hearing aids at home unless I have to, so once the weekend arrives, they are off from Friday to Monday morning.

I had not long been home, cleaned up and put some food on, the plan was to chill with a movie.

I took my hearing aids off and headed into the kitchen, noticing the doorbell flashing. I then went upstairs to look out of the window, just in case.

A man stood there, in a suit and holding a clipboard, so I quietly ignored him and returned to the kitchen.

A few minutes later, I saw him knocking on the window and ringing the doorbell again.

"Some people cannot take a hint," I thought. "Let's see what his problem is."

I went upstairs and put my implant processor on, and then went down and opened the door.

"Hello there," The man said. "How are you?"
"Fine," I replied. "How can I help?"
"Do you use broadband?" He asked. "Telephone?"
"I have broadband," I said. "Yes."
"Who is your supplier and what do you pay?" He asked.

I explained briefly who I was with and my monthly costs.

"I can get you a much better deal," He said. "More minutes and half the costs."
"I am not interested," I replied. "I am also busy so I need to go."
"Bear with me," He smiled. "I promise you will not be disappointed."
"Like I said," I rolled my eyes. "I have to go, I am happy with my supplier and have only recently signed up to them."
"How long is your contract?" He asked.
"Two years," I lied.

"You can pay to leave that contract," He said. "And sign up with us, you will get unlimited phone calls."

"They are no good to me," I said.

"Why not?" He asked.

"I am deaf," I said. "I don't use the phone."

"That is okay," He laughed. "You can let friends and family use it."

"No," I said. "Not interested."

"Give me one good reason why not," He said. "Go on."

"Because I am not," I replied. "I am happy with what I have and do not want to change."

"You can also get your mobile phone with us," He said. "A better deal than you currently have."

"I already have my mobile with my broadband supplier," I replied.

"Oh," He looked at his tablet. "Well, we can beat the price."

He showed me the prices on his tablet, over thirty pounds more than what I was currently paying.

"That is more than I pay now," I said.

"But you get free calls," He added.

"Again," I sighed. "No good to me."

"What will it take for you to change your mind?" He asked confidently.

"Nothing," I said. "Goodbye."

I closed the door and went back to cooking, leaving my implant in for the movie I had planned.

Twenty minutes later, the doorbell went again, so I went and opened it, and met with the same man from earlier.

"Have we met before?" He asked me.

"Are you winding me up today or something?" I asked. "Would you like me to call the police and ruin your day?"

"No need to be like that," He said. "I am only doing my job."

"Would you like to buy a broken lawnmower?" I asked him.

"Not particularly no," He said looking at me in confusion.

"Why not?" I asked. "It is very good and quiet."

"I am not interested in a broken lawnmower," He scoffed. "Why on earth are you trying to sell me a lawnmower?"

"Apologies," I said. "Considering you are being annoying and trying to flog me something I didn't want, I thought I would try the same."

At this point, the neighbour came out and started having a go at him. The police arrived sometime later after several complaints regarding the salesman trying to push an elderly couple into getting the deal because theirs was going out of action.

Nowadays, I rarely open the door unless I know who it is.

The pleasures of being deaf and not hearing the doorbell. (I turned off the flasher)

Deaf People Charity

It was slap bang in the middle of summer and very hot. I had just done some spring cleaning and had a cool shower. I came down to chill out with a game, ice cold beers. I had a friend over later in the day for a movie marathon and pizza.

The doorbell went as I put the game on and thought it was probably my friend as they liked to show up early, it was a couple of hours which I thought was odd.

I opened the door and a heavily built man stood there. Holding a folder in his hand, a rucksack over his back and his t-shirt were wet from the heavy sweat. He was bald and his head raw from the scorching sun, he had a goatee, well maintained.

"Hello there sir," He said. "How are you today?"
"Fine thanks," I said. "You?"
"Very well, thanks for asking," He said. "Enjoying the hot weather?" He sighed.
"Yes," I said. "How can I help?" I asked.

I didn't click on at first who he was or what he wanted.

"I am doing some research and hopefully finding some support for a charity I work with," He said. "May I have a few minutes?"

35

I am always happy to listen, just to see what he had to say and considering he was doing this in this weather, what was the harm?

"Sure," I said.

He opened his folder, showing me a photograph of children.

"The charity I work for is aimed at helping deaf children from backgrounds in poor communities, children that wouldn't normally get the help they so desperately need," He explained. "This involves help with communication, education and technology needs."

At this point, I realised that he hadn't noticed that I was deaf, my implant was covered by my long hair and I could understand him perfectly.

"Do you know sign language by any chance?" He asked.
"No," I lied.

I knew a little, not enough to communicate fully, but understood a fair amount.

"Let me show you some," He said.

He then attempted to badly sign, with no emotion and no sense. I let him do this for a while, pretending to be interested.

"Do you have any idea what I said?" He asked me, with a grin on his face.
"Absolute gibberish," I replied.
"No," he said. "That is what you call British Sign Language."
"No," I said. "I happen to be profoundly deaf."
"I don't think so," he laughed nervously.
"Why not?" I said.
"You are not deaf," He said.
"Why are you so sure?" I asked.
"Because you don't sign and your speech is normal," He chuckled. "That is how I know."
"Well you clearly haven't got a clue," I replied.

I showed him my implant processor.

"Oh," He said. "You should have told me."

"So you wouldn't attempt to scam me?" I said as I took my phone out of my pocket and took a photo of him.

"Why are you taking a photo of me?" He asked, slightly annoyed.

"To report you," I said.

"I am legit," He said, putting his things into his bag.

"Then you have nothing to worry about," I replied. "But I know for a fact, you cannot sign."

"It's a different kind of sign language," He said. "Universal."

"Nice try," I said. "Going to contact the police now."

I closed the door and watched him through the peephole having a meltdown. He rang the door a couple of times and hung around.

I reported him but never heard anything back, but the worrying thing is how much money did he make out of people who believed him.

Foreign student Scam

I had just been into town and was on my way home back to my aunt when I lived there, as I crossed the road a young woman came up to me, asking where a certain road was. I showed her where we were and then had a brief conversation.

I popped into the local fish and chip shop to get my aunt some lunch and then made my way back.

"Hello!" I called out to let her know I was in the house. "Dinner is served!"

"Hello David," My aunt appeared from the living room. "I have some news for you."

"Anything exciting?" I asked curiously.

"A nice young lady came to the door," She said. "Ever so pretty."

"Okay?" I said, wondering why.

She had a habit of trying to set me up with ladies, especially ones who came to the house.

37

"She was deaf," My aunt said. "And was selling some drawings."

"Oh right," I nodded.

"She couldn't speak and showed me a note," She replied. "I told her to come back, so you can have a look and buy some for me?"

"Do you want them?" I asked.

"Not really," She said. "But it helps the poor girl as she is struggling to find a job."

"Bit odd," I said. "Will have a look."

"She is a student from Poland," My aunt said, taking the fish and chips from me. "Her art is ever so good."

We sat down for dinner and then the doorbell rang. I opened the door and the girl from earlier asking for directions stood there, looking down at the floor and holding up a note that said, 'I a deaf student, no hearing, please help'.

"You seemed to hear okay earlier," I said. "We had a conversation and everything."

The girl looked up.

"Not understand," She said.

"Stop lying," I said. "Your English was fine earlier, or does it change when you go into scam mode?"

She panicked and turned, walking away in a hurry.

"You are on camera," I said. "If I see you again I will contact the police."

She gave me the two-finger salute and ran off, dropping some of the pictures as she disappeared around the block.

Have to say the pictures were very good, not sure if they were hers, but if they were, no idea why she was putting on an act.

"Who was it?" My aunt asked.

"The deaf girl," I said.

"And?" She asked in the middle of biting into a large chip.

"She was a scammer," I said. "Wasn't deaf at all."

"What?!" She banged her fork down in annoyance. "Why do people do that?"

"Because people suck," I said. "Wonder how many people she has conned with that act."

"What did she say?" She asked.

"Gave me two fingers and ran away," I laughed as I put the pictures in front of her. "Here you go, some freebies."

She was so annoyed that she put them in the bin.

DEAF AND DUMB

It was a wet and dull Saturday and I had just arrived at a book event in London, someone on Twitter had invited me along, telling me to bring some copies of my book. The Frustrations of being Deaf, part one. She had paid for a stall and asked if I wanted to go half, to showcase our books.

Had never attended anything like it, due to the fact I get nervous talking to strangers about my work. But I thought, just go for it, what do I have to lose?

I arrived to sign in, standing behind several people, only to find I was not on the list, and to make matters worse, the friend from Twitter had cancelled.

"Reasons for attending?" The man behind the desk asked.
"Got invited along," I replied.
"Author or reader?" He asked.
"Both," I said.
"What is that?" He pointed to my head. "Not seen a headset like that before."
"It's an implant processor," I said. "I am deaf."
"Oh," The man nodded in interest. "I would never have known."
"Hide it well," I smiled.
"Are you running a book stall?" He asked.
"I was going to join someone," I said. "But she has cancelled."
"Sorry to hear that," He said. "Do you know the stall number?"
"Thirty-two," I said looking through my phone.
"That was cancelled yesterday," He said. "Unfortunately has been given to someone else."
"Not a problem," I said. "I'll just have to chase my money!" I laughed.
"There is a generic stall where you can leave your books if you wish," He looked at the books in my hands. "If it helps, we have a disability stall at the end of the room, we have three authors there today."
"Thanks," I said, just about to walk through.
"Three pounds please," He said.
"What?" I was confused, after losing forty pounds to a stall I didn't get.
"Three pounds to enter," He said pointing to the sign on the desk.
"Expensive visit," I smiled, handing him the money.

I walked around the event, chatting to various people as I made my way towards the stall at the end of the room, where two people were. A woman leaning against the wall holding a cup of coffee and a man in a wheelchair.

"Afternoon," I said, checking my watch. "How is it going?"

"Slow," the man said. "But not too bad, I see you have bought some books?" He said.

"No," I laughed. "I was supposed to have a stall, but got let down, or scammed, not sure which."

"That sucks," He shook his head.

"How long have you had the implant?" The woman asked, stepping forward.

"About six years," I said. "The best decision I ever made."

"I am Kerri," She said holding out her hand. "This is Steve."

"Nice to meet you both," I said.

"I am registered blind," Kerri said. "And neurodiverse," Kerri said. "Depression and dyslexia too."

"What she means is she is a crazy cow," Steve said.

"I guess you can see some things?" I said.

"Shapes and lights," Kerri said. "Much better if I am closer, and the glasses help a tad."

"Well you noticed the implant," I said.

"Annoying LED on the top," She smiled.

"I am in a wheelchair in case you are wondering," Steve chuckled.

"No we didn't notice," Kerri said. "Attention seeker."

"Paralysed from the lower chest down," He said. "Boy racer on my street when I was a kid."

"Serves you right for playing in the road," Kerri scoffed.

"He hit a Royal Mail post box before me," Steve said. "And I was on the path outside my house."

"Sorry to hear that," I said.

A middle-aged man walked over to the stall, with several books in a plastic bag.

"Hello," He said. "Is this a science fiction stall?"

He was kidding, but not very well.

"Yes," Kerri said. "We are the realistic X-Men."

"Oh," The man said curiously.

"This is what mutation looks like," she nodded. "Blind, no sonar skills or anything."

"I am deaf," I replied. "Crap genetics, but now part cyborg."

"I thought I was immune to cars," Steve grinned. "Turns out I am not and my spine got squished."

The man looked ever so uncomfortable.

"We are kidding," I said. "We aren't X-Men."

"So tell me about your books," He said curiously.

"Mine is an autobiography," Steve said. "I got fed up with constantly telling my story and decided to write it."

"Interesting," The man said. "How about you?" He looked at Kerri.

"Dating woes," Kerri said. "And depression woes."

"And you?" The man looked me up and down. "Are you disabled?"

"Yes," I said. "Allergic to people."

He looked at me, unimpressed.

"I am deaf," I said. "My books are comedy based on true stories."

"Oh," The man said. "Really?"

"Yes," I replied.

"You don't seem deaf," He said curiously.

"I deal with it well," I said. "Implant helps."

"So how long have you been deaf and dumb?" He asked outright.

Steve and Kerri looked at each other, and then at the man.

"What?" I said, a little shocked.

"I said," The man raised his voice. "How long have you been deaf and dumb."

"You do realise that using the word dumb is offensive," Kerri said.

"No, it isn't," The man said. "It's an expression to describe deaf people."

"You are wrong," I said. "Deaf and dumb is an old expression and also a degrading way of describing someone who is deaf and mute," I sighed. "Or most commonly used, deaf without speech."

"I think you are wrong," He chuckled. "I am going to google it."

"Go for it," I said. "Do you have Google for idiots installed on your phone?"

He ignored me and started searching online, and the grin on his face slowly disappeared.

"I apologise," He said. "Let me rephrase, how long have you been deaf without speech?"

Again, I looked at him in surprise.

"How long have you been stupid?" I asked.
"What did you say to me?" He demanded.
"Nothing," I said. "I am deaf without speech remember?"

Kerri laughed while Steve rolled his eyes and shook his head.

"You know he can talk right?" Steve said.
"Yes," The man said, suddenly realising. "Oh, I get you."
"Do you?" Steve said.
"What is your book about?" The man asked me.
"It's about a deaf author that invites someone that insulted him back to his cabin, ties him up and goes all Anne Wilkes on his ankles," I said grinning.
"Loved that book," Steve said.
"I am going to go," The man said, turning around slowly and walking away before glancing back.

A woman walked over, one of the organisers.

"Everything okay?" She asked.
"Yes," Steve said. "Just that guy giving Dave grief for being deaf and dumb."
"Oh that is the incorrect term," She said. "Should be deaf and mute."
"He struggled with the fact I wasn't actually mute," I said. "Although, I can think of a fair amount of people that wish I was."

I ended up giving all my books away, mainly to the nicer people I had met and shared stories with.

Next time, I am stocking up on copies of Misery for the idiots.

DEAF IN BRUGES

Back in 2003, my aunt booked a day trip to Bruges to do something different, and she wanted to treat me to a day out.

Not being a fan of coach or ferry trips, I asked why she wanted to go, however, she just said she wanted breakfast and lunch in Bruges as she had been there before and enjoyed it.

We arrived at the pick-up point and she had asked me for the tenth time if I had my passport, probably to wind me up because I had got to the edge of the road before realising I had left it on the counter, along with my wallet.

The coach pulled up and there were several of us waiting to get on. My aunt was chatting away with this older woman and her daughter who had downs, she knew them both well and it was my first time meeting them.

> "This is David," My aunt said introducing me.
> "Dave," I corrected her.
> "Your birth certificate says David," She said smugly.
> "Was he christened David?" The woman asked.
> "No," My aunt said. "His parents never had him christened."
> "Just as well," I added. "Otherwise I would have been christened David Alice!"
> "Oh behave!" My aunt said.

We got onto the coach and it smelt of damp and cheap air freshener, it was going to be a bloody long day.

The organiser went from seat to seat, checking people's tickets and passports. He approached me and before I could speak, my aunt chipped in.

> "He is deaf," She said. "Make sure you face him and speak clearly."
> "Nice to meet you deaf," He said with a grin.
> "Very funny," I said, looking at my aunt and shaking my head. "He doesn't need to know that."
> "I am only helping," She said.

"Is this your mum?" The man asked.

"My warden," I replied. "She lets me out once a month."

"Bloody cheek!" She scoffed. "I am his great Aunt," She said. "His grandmother's sister."

"Are you sure?" The man said curiously. "You seem way too young!"

I laughed and she glared at me.

"Will we be going to the duty-free?" She asked.

"On the way back yes," The man said. "What is your poison?"

At this point, I was curious as she had said nothing about duty-free.

"What are you going to the duty-free for?" I asked.

"Never you mind!" She said and laughed.

"Oh," I said in excitement. "What are you buying me!?"

"Nothing," She said. "You get breakfast if you are good."

"Charming," I said. "I would prefer vodka."

"Tough," She replied. "You don't drink vodka."

"I do," I nodded.

"Well you are not having any," She said.

"Better do as you are told," The man said to me. "It's not worth the hassle."

"Behave," She warned me.

"Could I see your passports?" He said. "Need to check them over before we leave."

I handed my passport, watching as my aunt was searching through her handbag for hers.

"Not forgotten it have you?" The man asked.

"Especially after the nagging you gave me before we left the house!" I said, shaking my head.

"Don't be rude!" She said, finally pulling out her passport and handing it to the man who opened it and checked it.

"Have you seen the date of birth?" He said. "They got it wrong!"

I rolled my eyes, handing him mine.

"Lovely photo!" He laughed. "Were you stoned or half asleep?"

"Cannot remember," I said. "Probably tired."

"He always looks like that," My aunt said as she took the passport from the man.

"You will need to get that renewed next year," He said.

"Not planning on travelling," I said.

"You never know," He smiled. "Your aunt may drag you on another booze run!"

We ended up playing Rummy on the journey to Bruges, and I was getting hungry despite eating before we left. When we arrived we stopped off for a late breakfast at this amazing café, only because I could smell the waffles before we got there.

"Good morning," The waitress said. "What would you like?"

My aunt looked at me, waiting for me to say something.

"Sorry," I said. "Could you repeat that?"

"What would you like?" She asked again.

I could not lipread her and she had a strong accent.

"Do you mind?" I looked at my aunt.

"Sorry," She said. "My boy is deaf," She stuck her tongue out. "What would you like?"

"You go first," I said, looking through the menu.

"Do you want me to order for you?" My aunt asked.

"No I do not," I said. "Don't trust you!"

"How long have you been deaf?" She asked me.

"Did you ask how long I have been deaf?" I said.

She nodded.

"About twenty years," I said. "Went deaf at seven."

"Do you know sign?" She asked.

"DO I know what?" I said.

"Sign," She said imitating sign language.

"No," I said. "Never needed to learn but would like to."

46

She smiled.

We both ordered our food and sat for a while, chatting and drinking refills of coffee and tea, something I regretted later.

Later that evening, we returned to the coach collection point, to find the coach wasn't there.

"Have we missed it?" She said looking at me. "Did you get the time wrong?"
"No," I said looking at my watch. "It's four o'clock!"
"Did you listen when he spoke to you?" She asked.
"You were there too," I laughed. "Were you not listening?"
"Cheek!" She said. "I am sure they said four."
"They did," I nodded. "They will be along soon."
"What if we miss the coach?" She said in panic.
"Stay in a hotel for the evening, then book a ferry back," I said. "Or a train."
"I have no clean clothes," She said.
"Neither do I," I laughed. "The coach will be along soon."

We waited a few minutes and the coach pulled up, slowly turning, and stopping in front of us.

"You two are early," The man said looking at his watch. "Well, a few minutes."
"My aunt was so sure we missed the bus," I said laughing.
"Don't tell tales!" She said.
"You can get on if you want," He said. "We will leave in fifteen minutes for the duty-free stop-off."
"How long will we be there?" My aunt asked.
"Half an hour," He said. "Should give everyone a chance."
"Are you going to get anything?" She asked.
"No," I said. "Don't need anything?"

We arrived at the duty-free and my aunt got the tobacco for her brother while I waited outside with a cup of coffee that I got from the café.

"Got everything?" I asked my aunt as she walked over, a pack of rolling tobacco under her arm and a bottle of vodka in the other hand.

"Got you a present," She said holding up the vodka.

"Oh!" I said in excitement. "I'll have that next weekend!"

"It has to last you a year!" She warned me and handed the bottle to me. "Carry this, it's heavy."

"Did they not have any bags?" I asked. "Tight sods."

"The driver said he has bags," She said and rolled her eyes. "Were you not listening?"

"I might leave you here if you keep it up," I said. "Let you walk back."

"I have the passports," She said, poking out her tongue.

We walked back towards the coach, talking about the day we had and as she approached the kerb, she stumbled and fell forward into the road.

"Shit!" I said. "Are you okay?!"

She got to her knees, laughing.

"Help me up," She said.

I put down the vodka and coffee on the edge of the curb, noticing the coach driver hurrying towards us. I got hold of her arm, gently trying to lift her but she couldn't stand up fully.

"Have you broken something?" I asked.

She shook her head, laughing and trying to talk.

"Hold on mate," The coach driver ran over. "You are standing on her handbag strap!" He pointed.

Without realising, I had stood on the handbag strap, which was looped over her neck, and trying to lift her at the same time, strangling her.

"Sorry!" I said and moved back, helping her stand along with the help of the coach driver.

"Are you okay?" He said. "Sure you haven't broken anything?"

"Only my neck," She laughed, coughing slightly.

"Sorry!" I said, feeling bad.

"It was an accident," She said. "You couldn't hear me," She then looked at me curiously. "Could you?"

"No," I said noticing her knee was bleeding. "You have hurt your knee."

48

"It's a scratch," She said scoffing.

"Let's get on the bus, my colleague can dress that for you," The driver said.

We got on the bus and the driver's assistant dressed my aunt's knee while we got underway, making our way to the ferry.

"Oh no!" My aunt said.

"What?" I asked. "Did it hurt?"

"I have sat on the tobacco!" She realised, shifting to one side to reveal the crushed pack.

"Oh crap," I said. "I left my coffee and vodka on the side of the road!"

Lucky for me, someone a few seats down had found the vodka and on overhearing, let me have it back. The coffee however was a lost cause.

DEAF SPEAK

After a few days of having issues with my throat, I booked an appointment with my doctor's surgery to try and get to the bottom of it.

I turned up and booked an emergency appointment, told to sit down and wait until I was called. I had spoken to the receptionist, letting her know that I was profoundly deaf and would need someone to point me out, especially as they didn't have a visual system.

An hour or so later, I was getting uncomfortable and frustrated, my throat was raw and sore.

I looked up at the reception and saw the receptionist, calling me over, so I got up and walked over, hoping it was good news.

A man was standing at the counter, looking stressed.

"Could you translate for me," She said.
"Translate what?" I asked in confusion.
"What is he saying?" She said. "We are not very good with deaf speak."
"Deaf speak?" I said and looked at the man who signed to me, asking if I was deaf.
"You mean sign language," I said. "Not deaf speak."
"I couldn't think of the words," She laughed.
"Right," I said, unimpressed. "I don't sign."
"But you are deaf," She said. "Or was you telling me fibs?"
"I am deaf," I replied. "I don't sign and don't need to."
"I am confused," She laughed. "So you cannot translate?"

I looked at the man and speaking carefully and trying to remember how to sign, I asked what the problem was.

He explained that his prescription was wrong and that he needed the correct one from his doctor.

I explained to the receptionist, who then wanted me to confirm his details.

"Do you have a notepad?" I asked. "And a pen, rather than this poor guy share his private details with a stranger?"

"I do," She smiled. "I just thought all deaf people stuck together."

"Do ignorant people stick together?" I asked.

"I have no idea," She said looking at me curiously.

A woman walked in, standing next to the man.

"Everything okay?" She asked.

"I was asked if I understood deaf speak," I said and rolled my eyes.

"Deaf speak?" She scoffed. "Really?" She looked up at the receptionist. "What an earth was going through your head?"

"I didn't know what they called it," She said.

"British Sign Language?" She said. "There is no such thing as deaf speak!" She said.

"Do you know my dad?" She looked at me.

"No," I replied. "The receptionist called me over."

"Thank you for your help," she said. "I am here now so I will help my dad with the deaf speak!" She said in sarcasm.

I sat back down, looking up every so often and wondering how much longer I was going to wait. After an hour, I got up and walked over to the reception.

"Could you tell me how much longer?" I asked.

"Waiting times are an hour," She said to me bluntly.

"I have been here two hours," I replied.

A doctor looked up from behind the counter.

"Mr Blackwell?" He said. "We called but didn't get a response."

"I asked reception to let me know," I said. "I am deaf."

"I forgot," she said. "Sorry about that."

"Funny thing to forget after the whole deaf-speak incident," I replied. "Sounds to me like you had the hump."

"Deaf speak?" The doctor said looking confused.

"I am going to go to accident and emergency," I said. "They won't treat me like an idiot."

51

"If you would like to wait half an hour," The doctor said. "I will try and fit you in."

"It's fine," I replied. "I will go elsewhere, maybe they have deaf speakers at the hospital?" I walked out smiling and made my way to the hospital.

I only waited for half an hour, strangely enough, no deaf speak was available.

DEBT COLLECTORS

I had just got home from work and was putting away some shopping, getting ready to cook some dinner. My implant battery had died, and I wasn't bothered until I noticed the doorbell flashing.

Putting in a new battery, the doorbell went, followed by someone knocking on the door loudly and impatiently.

"Just a minute," I called out, turning off the hob and moving the frying pan.

I opened the door to find two men, one heavily built with black trousers, a black t-shirt and what looked like a stab vest with a camera mounted. The second man was shorter, slimmer, and older, wearing the same.

"Yes?" I said.
"Any reason why you didn't answer the door straight away?" He said. "We knew you were in."
"I am deaf," I replied. "Implant battery went."
"If you say so," He said.

The smaller man, looking at a clipboard tried to walk in, mumbling.

"Can I help you?" I said, holding the door firmly.
"We are here about an unpaid debt," He said. "We need to collect payment or procure goods to cover the cost of the dept."
"I think you have the wrong person," I replied.

He handed me a form, with my address however the name of the person was a resident who had left several years before. I had received various letters addressed to him and had a visit from another agency trying to track him down. However since, I had heard nothing more.

"That isn't me," I replied. "I have returned the letters back to you about this."
"You will be surprised how many people say that," The man scoffed. "We require payment today."
"As I have just said," I said. "That isn't my debt."

The man said something to his colleague who laughed.

"Wait here and I will get my identification," I said.
"Can we come in?" He asked.
"No," I said. "I will be back in a moment."

I closed the door and he put his foot in it, preventing me.

"Could you not do that?" I replied.
"I know what you are planning to do," He said. "You are going to lock us out."
"I am getting my wallet," I said.
"Let us in," He asked.
"No," I replied. "I will be back."

I closed the door, however, didn't lock it properly and they both walked in.

"My colleague will start recording goods," He said. "If you get your wallet, we can make payment if you have it."
"What part of what I said do you not understand?" I replied. "I am not the person on that form!"
"We will need to see some identification," He said.
"That is why I asked you to wait!" I snapped.

The larger man was about to walk upstairs.

"If you go upstairs," I warned him. "You better be prepared to be sued."

He ignored me, making his way into the living room.

"Television," He wrote down the details. "Laptop computer," be bent down, picking it up.

I got my mobile from my pocket, texted a friend and asked them to call the police for me, giving them the basics.

"Who are you texting?" The man asked.
"Police," I replied. "You have pushed your way into my home."

"We are waiting for you to produce Identification," He said.

"Go back outside and I will get it," I said. "I do not trust you to be left alone," I indicated to his colleague. "Look at him!"

"Go and get your identification and we will wait here," He said.

"No," I replied. "I want you both outside the front door and I will then get my wallet."

"Not happening," He said.

"Fine," I laughed. "I will let the police deal with it."

I sat down and refused to speak to him, putting the video recorder on my mobile phone.

Within ten minutes, the police arrived, a male and female hurrying in. I met them in the hallway.

"Hi," I said. "They both pushed their way into my house and they have the wrong person."

"We have asked for identification," The man said. "And he refused."

"Asked them to wait outside," I said. "He refused and pushed his way in, and I didn't want to leave them alone."

"We would have waited," He said. "But he was ignoring or avoiding our questions.

"You started recording my property and touched it," I replied. "That is why I didn't trust you."

"You also avoided answering the door," He grinned.

"As I have said, I am deaf," I said, biting my tongue. "But then again you have selective hearing."

"Could I see the form?" The male officer said.

The man handed it to him.

"Are you Pakistani sir?" the officer asked me.

"No," I replied. "Thought that would be obvious."

The officer looked at the man.

"Could you wait outside please?" The officer asked the man.

"I would rather wait inside," The man said.

"Well I am asking you to wait outside, we will confirm this gentleman's identification," He said.

"And if he is who you say he is, we will allow you access."

Both of the men left, waiting on the drive as the female officer closed the door and locked it. I then went upstairs to find my wallet and passport, coming down a few seconds later.

"Here," I handed both to the officer.

"This is clearly a case of mistaken identity," The officer said examining both.

"I would have shown them," I said. "But they pushed in."

"Not acceptable," He said.

All three of us went outside and the officer explained to the man that the person they were looking forward to is no longer at the address.

"Do you have a forwarding address?" The man asked me.

"No," I replied. "I have only been here a year and a half."

"Can I have your landlord's details?" He asked.

"Why," I asked. "So you can harass her?"

"No," He laughed. "We want to confirm details."

"I'll let her know," I replied. "I will also be making a complaint against your company for the attitude and unprofessionalism today."

"We did nothing wrong," The man said, looking me up and down. "If you had been cooperative."

"You pushed your way into the property," The female officer replied. "And if you needed to, you would require police presence."

"We did request the police," The larger man said.

"What is the number?" She asked. "They would have given you a number."

"I forget," The man said.

"Talking out of his arse," I said. "I am going to send an amazing and long email, as well as some free social media coverage for you."

"You are not allowed to do that," The man said.

"You pushed into my home and treated me like crap," I said. "Regardless of the fact I told you I was deaf, you ignored me."

"You don't look deaf," The man argued.

"Do I look Pakistani?" I asked. "Have to say, you look just how you are."

"Which is what?" The man asked.

"Ignorant," I said bluntly. "Now get lost please."

"Could you confirm your full name and date of birth?" The man asked.

"No," I replied. "Do I need to press charges for you to take a hint?"

56

"Please leave the property," The male officer said, leading them towards the front door.

The men left and the police took further details from me, stating they would contact the company and warn them of the procedures they should follow.

A few months later, another company visited regarding a three-thousand-pound unpaid bill from a telephone company, a much better and more professional encounter.

I got an email from the debt collector company, claiming it was a simple mistake and that the two men would have refresher training.

I left them a lovely review online, considering I wasn't a customer, lucky them.

DISABLED PERSON ASSISTANCE

I was in a department store getting some clothes, when I found a shirt I liked but couldn't find my size on the rack so I decided to see if they had any additional stock.

I queued at customer service for a few minutes.

Someone tapped me on the shoulder and I turned around.

"Daydreaming?" The woman said and pointed.
"Sorry?" I asked.
"Til at the end," The woman said.
"Thanks," I said and made my way to the till, met with an assistant with a beaming smile.
"Good morning sir," She said. "How can I help?"
"Was wondering if you had this in a forty-four chest?" I said, handing the shirt to her.
"Let me see if I can find out," She said and then said something else which I didn't catch.
"Sorry, could you repeat that?" I asked.
"I asked if you needed help with anything else?" She said, then noticing my implant. "Oh, are you deaf?" She said, raising her voice and emphasising her words.
"Yes," I nodded. "But just speak normally."
"Okay," She nodded, not changing anything. "Let me find out if someone from the stores can have a look for you."
"Thanks," I said and stood back as she approached the intercom system.
"Assistance required from stores for a disabled customer at the customer service counter!" Her voice boomed on the intercom, she repeated it twice.

Eyes were on me, people looking me up and down, probably wondering what disability I had.

"Oh bloody hell," I muttered under my breath.

The girl then looked at me with a smile.

"Someone will be here shortly," She said loudly.

"Thanks," I said, slightly embarrassed and wondering whether to make a quick getaway, but I liked the shirt.

A few minutes passed and a woman walked up to the counter, speaking to the girl who pointed to me.

"Hello there sir," She said. "How can I help you?" She looked me up and down.
"I was wondering if you had this shirt in forty-four chest?" I said.
"I can have a look," she said. "What is your disability if you don't mind me asking?"
"Deaf," I said.
"Okay sir," she raised her voice.
"Just speak normally," I said. "No need to talk loudly."
"I have a deaf aunt," She said, emphasising her words. "Age-related deafness, so I know how to speak to deaf people."
"We are all different," I said. "I am a natural one from the wild."

She looked at me strangely.

"What do you mean?" She asked.
"I went deaf at a young age," I said. "However I am implanted."
"Implanted how?" She said.
"SO they can track me," I said grinning.
"You are winding me up!" She scoffed. "Is that an ear implant?"
"Cochlear implant," I said. "Gives me hearing and I rely on lip-reading to communicate."
"So what shall I do?" She said.
"Speak normally," I replied. "If I miss anything, I will ask you to repeat it."
"Understood," She said. "Let me go and check this for you."

I stood around for a while, and she never came back, so I went to pay for the goods I had and was back with the same girl as before.

"Did you find everything, sir?" She asked.
"Yes," I said. "Although that woman went off to check the shirts and never turned up."
"Oh," She said. "Would you like me to find her?"
"No it is okay," I said. "Just these."
"I don't mind," She said smiling. "I am happy to put out an announcement."

"No," I said. "I have had enough fun for the day, so just these."

As the girl ran things through and slowly packed them, someone called out.

"Sir?!" The voice echoed. "Excuse me!"

The girl pointed to someone behind me.

I turned around and saw the woman from earlier, holding up a couple of shirts.

"Hi sir," She shouted. "We don't have a forty-four, however, we do have a forty and a forty-eight?"
"No thanks," I said.
"Are you sure?" She asked.
"I am," I said. "And I think the entire store is too."

I paid and left, not a fan of being the centre of attention in a department store.

DISABLED PERSON

It was the weekend and I had popped into work to get my mobile phone after leaving it behind the day before.

I made my way through towards the workshop, stopping in the shop to get a bottle of water and bumping into one of the porters I had known for several years, and we had a conversation.

"Are you okay there love?" He said looking at me.
"Who are you calling love?" I said to him. "You want a hug or something?"
"Not you!" He said pushing me gently to the side. "Hello."

A little old lady stood there, holding a handbag in one hand and a letter in the other.

"Could you tell me where this is?" She said holding up the letter.

The porter took the letter and read it, smiling and nodding.

"Up one floor and at the end of the corridor," He said.
"I can take you there if you like," I said.
"Do you mind?" She asked. "That would be kind of you."

I led her to the lift and called it, standing by the door.

"How is your day going?" I asked her.
"It is okay," She said. "I have done my shopping and now visiting my son."
"Hope he is on the road to recovery," I said with a smile.
"He is a simple boy," She said shaking her head. "Was never right from the day he was born, very different to his sister."
"Sorry to hear that," I replied.
"He was always special," She nodded.

The lift arrived and I let her get in, pressing the button.

"Are you visiting someone?" She asked.

"Sorry," I said, the noise of the automated message blocking out her voice.

"What for?" She said.

"I didn't hear what you said," I said. "Could you repeat it?"

"Oh," She noticed my hearing aid. "You are disabled."

"Profoundly deaf," I said. "What did you say?"

"I asked if you were visiting someone?" She said, talking slower and clearer.

"I work here," I said. "Left my phone behind last night so I popped in to get it."

"Do you not work weekends?" She said.

"No," I replied. "Sometimes I do to catch up, but not today."

How long have you worked here?" She asked.

"About sixteen years now," I said.

"It's very nice of the hospital to give a disabled person a job," She said. "I hope they don't give you anything too hard to do, we don't want you making mistakes now do we."

I laughed, shocked but found it funny.

"What do they have you doing?" She asked. "Portering? Cleaning?"

The lift arrived and the door opened, I let her walk out and then slowly followed.

"I am an engineer," I said.

"Really?" She said in surprise. "They let you do that?"

"Yes," I replied. "Done it a while, so."

"Oh," She nodded. "Maybe my son could get a job doing what you do?"

"Maybe," I said. "Tell him to apply."

I showed her where the ward was and then made my way back downstairs, bumping into the porter again.

"That was quick," He said.

"She had a bloody cheek," I scoffed.

"Why?" He asked me.

"She said, It's very nice of the hospital to give a disabled person a job," I mimicked her. "I hope they don't give you anything too hard to do, we don't want you making mistakes now do we."

62

"Well," He said. "Sounds like she knows you."

"Said the guy that escaped the asylum!" I said.

"Well, how did you get your job?" He asked curiously.

"Told my manager I was bored and she recommended I go in there," I said. "Been trapped ever since!" I walked away laughing.

DOESN'T MATTER

My BIGGEST pet hate is when someone speaks to me and I struggle to understand, maybe two or three times, and they give up with a simple "Oh it doesn't matter." So why talk to me in the first place?

I was queuing up at the checkout at a supermarket on the way home, it was a Friday evening so I had planned to make a Chinese, a few drinks, and a movie.

It was moving slowly, with lots of empty checkouts so clearly had staffing issues.

I was on my phone when the man behind the checkout thumped on the conveyor.

"Is this yours?" He pointed to the shopping I had laid out.
"Yes," I nodded.
"Need a bag?" He asked.
"No thanks," I said pulling one out of my pocket.
"Cool," He said and went back to serving the woman in front of me.

A few minutes passed and the woman behind me was starting to get on my nerves, talking loudly on the phone and bumping her trolley into me.

"I can't move any further," I said to her. "Someone in front of me."
"Okay," She said shaking her head in confusion. "I never asked."
"Oh I thought you were dropping hints by nudging me with the trolley," I said.
"Sorry," She said. "It's on a slope."

I turned around, rolling my eyes at the so-called slope.

"You need any bags?" The man behind the checkout asked again as the person in front of me moved away and I walked to the end.
"No," I said. "You already asked that."
"Did I?" He said curiously. "I see so many people I lose track."
"It's cool," I said.

He passed the things down and I packed, wondering why he was moving at a super slow speed, worried the chicken would go off.

He said something to me when I was looking down, and over the noise, I didn't understand him.

"What was that?" I asked.

He said it again, but I struggled.

"Sorry, can you repeat that?" I asked.

He then waved me away and said...

"Doesn't matter," He said bluntly.

I was a bit taken aback, as well as annoyed.

"So why did you ask?" I said. "If it doesn't matter."

"I am busy," he said. "Cannot mess around if you are not bothered to listen."

"It's not the fact I am not bothered," I said. "I am deaf."

"Of course you are," He said chuckling.

I looked at him in amazement.

"You think I wear this as a fashion statement?" I asked.

"Bluetooth," He said. "Loads of people have them."

"Not this one," I pointed to my processor. "It's worth more than a small car."

A woman walked over to the counter with a "Supervisor" Badge.

"Hi, is everything okay?" she asked.

The till operator turned around and spoke to her.

"What seems to be the problem, sir?" She asked me.

"No problem," I said. "I asked him to repeat something and he was rude about it."

"I was not rude," he scoffed.

"I told you I was deaf and you responded with," I paused. "Of course you are."

"Well you heard that," He said, almost mockingly.

"Do you lip-read?" The woman asked me.

"Yes," I said. "I struggled to understand him due to the background noise.

"What did you ask?" She asked the man.

"Nothing," He said.

"Well you must have asked something?" she smiled. "I can relay the question."

"I asked if he had identification," He said pointing to the alcohol I had purchased.

"I do," I said. "I am in my forties, but more than happy to supply identification."

"Not required," She said. "I will give you a discount for your trouble."

"Thanks," I said.

"Typical," The man scoffed.

"Could you leave please," The supervisor said. "Go and take a break, you clearly need it."

The man sulked off and the woman served me, giving me a discount and apologising for the attitude.

Some people get embarrassed, and usually as a result become rude or ignorant, but at the end of the day, I didn't ask to be deaf.

EYE TEST

I started to struggle with my eyes a few years ago, probably the constant writing and having the television on in the background. My right eye is bad enough due to the damage from a squint repair, I am pretty sure the doctor had the shakes. I was getting headaches and tiredness whenever reading or writing, so I booked an appointment with an optician, something I don't take lightly.

I knew it was going to be an awkward visit when I got to reception and the girl behind the reception had a mask on.

"Hi," I said. "I have an appointment, Dave Blackwell."

She stood up, said something, and then walked away. I stood around for a couple of minutes, and another woman turned up, wearing a mask. She said something, I think.

"I am deaf," I said. "Do you mind lowering your mask so I can lipread?"

She shook her head and raised her voice.

"I cannot understand you," I said. "I have an appointment," I looked at my watch. "Now."

Another woman came over, not wearing a mask.

"How can I help," She said.
"I have an appointment," I said. "For an eye test and glasses."
"Could you go and sit over there," She pointed. "You will be called."
"Could someone let me know please," I said. "I am deaf and probably won't hear."
"I will let them know," She said.

Ten minutes passed and I heard my name yelled out, so loud I think the people on the floor below also heard.

"Daydreaming?" The woman said with a smile.
"Deaf," I said.

"Oh sorry," she chuckled. "You should have said."

"I did," I said. "Couple of times."

She took me into the room, checked my eyes, and then explained how she needed to check the pressure. The room was fairly dark, which didn't do much for lipreading, so I struggled.

"Any questions?" She asked.

"So I look ahead and keep my eye still?" I asked.

"Yes," She said. "On the count of three, I will press the button, so you will feel a little rush of air."

"Okay thanks," I said.

I sat there, with my chin on the rest and looking directly at the light, waiting.

I heard her mumble something and moved, resulting in a rush of air on my nose.

"I said not to move!" She said.

"You also promised a countdown," I replied. "It's bad enough trying to lipread."

"Can you not turn your hearing aid up," She moaned. "Things would be so much better."

"It doesn't work like that," I said. "What do you do for blind people? Turn the lights up?"

She sat back, looking at me very unimpressed.

"Let's try again shall we?" She said.

I put my chin on the rest and didn't move a muscle until I felt both of my eyes tested.

If you think that was bad, the next woman, doing the fitting for glasses, had no patience! She wore a mask and wanted me to sit in the semi-dark, with a frame on my face checking if the letters were clear and easy to read, that was a long ten minutes!

By the time I had finished, I was knackered from the constant need to have to focus, because they didn't want to meet me halfway. I went and had a look at the frames, I had an idea of what I wanted, but the selection was good.

After a few minutes, one of the women came over, hovering behind me.

"Do you need help?" She asked.

"No I am good thanks, just trying to make up my mind," I said, holding a thin silver-rimmed frame.

"What about black?" She said. "They would match your hearing aid."

"Pass," I smiled.

"Did you get it from boots?" She asked.

"What?" I said. "The processor?"

"The hearing aid yes," She said. "We also do them."

"You won't have anything this good," I said.

"How are you so sure?" She questioned.

"Because this is a cochlear implant processor," I said. "Not a boots hearing aid."

"Oh," She said in surprise. "Can you hear anything with it?"

"Would be a waste of time wearing it if I couldn't," I said smiling.

"That is so cool," She nodded. "What about your other hearing aid," She said looking at my right ear. "That looks like a normal hearing aid."

"It is," I said. "And no I don't want to buy a hearing aid."

Eventually, she left me alone and I picked out the frames.

The whole experience will mean I will go elsewhere the next time I need glasses and talk about pain!

69

FLYING TOYS

Sometimes I think I am unlucky, clumsy too, but mainly just unlucky.

I was invited to a friend's for dinner and she had a little boy that was about four at the time, and ever so excited to show me everything he had.

He was playing with his toys when I was talking to his mother, drinking coffee.

"Dave!" He said in excitement and swung a rubber hammer at me, knocking the coffee clean out of my hand.

It went all over the grey carpet, missing my friend by inches.

She told him off and explained to him that I am deaf, and he needs to face me when he speaks to me.

I watched as he listened, the broken cup handle still in my hand.

He then came up to me with tons of questions about my hearing aids and became fascinated with the implant, lifting it on and off. After a while, he disappeared into the next room while my friend brought me a fresh coffee. We talked some more and he walked in, giggling and hiding something.

"What are you doing?" She asked him.

He then put a fridge magnet, the letter D on my implant and reduced his mother to hysterics.

"What is it?" I asked. "What did he put on my hearing aid?"
"D for?" She said.
"D for Dave!" The boy yelled in my ear and I could have sworn my eyes rolled like slot machines.
"Don't shout in his ear!" His mum said in between laughing. "You will hurt him!"

He looked at me curiously.

"Remember what I said?" She said to him.

"I know," He said and returned to playing with his toys.

We talked a little while and she went into the kitchen to sort out dinner, asking me to keep an eye on the boy.

"Dave!" He said.

"What?" I looked at him curiously.

He burst into giggles, hiding behind the armchair and I looked away.

"Dave!" He said and then hid.

"Who said that?!" I said, pretending to be shocked.

I looked away, glancing at my mobile.

"Dave!" He said again and hid.

"What!?" I looked up. "Who said that?!"

"I looked away for a minute, waiting for him to call me again.

"Dave!" He called out.

As I looked around, a toy car crashed into my face, and I saw stars, followed by a metallic taste in my mouth.

"Owch!" I yelped.

The boy fell to the floor, giggling.

My friend walked in just as my nose erupted, blood pouring down my face and into my hand as I stopped it from landing on the carpet.

"What happened?" She said. "Oh no," She looked at the boy, standing behind the sofa looking guilty. "Did you throw something at Dave?"

He nodded and giggled.

"That wasn't nice!" She said and then looked at me. "Sorry, he plays with his dad and he dives out of the way."

"It's okay," I said. "Got any tissue?"

I went into the toilet and sorted myself out, the bleeding stopped after a few minutes.

An hour or so later after having dinner, the boy was fascinated with the implant so I let him play with random magnets, sticking them on the processor.

"Come on you," She said. "Time to get ready for bed."

"Soon," he said.

"Better do what mummy said," I turned around, just as he went to put the letter F on my implant, poking me in the eye with it.

I swear I was on the set of Larry, Curly and Moe that day, sore eye and a sore nose. Practically beaten up all day by a four-year-old.

I saw him again a few years later, and he never laid a finger on me. He did, however, kick my butt at every game we played.

IMPLANT BATTERY WOES

The battery for my implant gives me at least nine hours of normal use, however, the more noise the less it runs.

I have three batteries for my implant and always make sure I have a spare on me, I can manage without it, however those around me panic when they realise.

I stopped in the coffee shop near the end of the day, I needed a strong coffee and there was also someone I really liked sitting near the window. I had finally built up the courage to speak to her.

I had spoken to her on several occasions, I struggled to lip-read her, however, practice makes perfect!

"Hi," I said. "Could I get you a coffee?" I asked her.

At this point, my implant battery decided to die, strangely enough with no warning. Usually, I get a series of beeps every fifteen minutes for a quarter of an hour. I also didn't have one on me, it was in my jacket in the workshop.

I went tried to speak to her, but couldn't understand what she was saying, and it got awkward.

"I will be back in a moment," I said, returning to the workshop to change the battery.

When I came back, she had gone and annoyingly, I hadn't seen her since.

Missing Battery

It was the weekend and I was spring cleaning, mainly due to losing two of my batteries. The remaining one was on a charge, and I wanted to watch a film. I looked high and low, checking my bag, jacket, and the usual spots.

I concluded that I had left one at work on my bench, however I was still unable to locate the third one.

I turned the house upside down, getting annoyed at myself for not looking after it. I double-checked all the usual places.

I used the half-charged battery and as I came downstairs, the washing machine was making an annoying clicking sound.

"Crap!" I said when I noticed the hearing aid battery clattering around in the washing machine, hitting the door every so often.

Luckily, I managed to stop the washing machine and retrieve it. Placing it in some dry packs for a day, and it works fine still.

Not a Battery

Before going out to meet a friend and see a film, I was rushing around to get ready and didn't quite check what I was doing. I put the spare battery in my top pocket and head out the door.

Had dinner, a long chat and then went into the cinema. Ten minutes into the film, my implant started beeping, indicating a flat battery, so I decided to change it there and then.

I reached into my pocket and took out the battery, removing my implant and then fiddling around in the darkness, trying to fit it.

That was when I realised I had picked up a USB stick, and not the battery. The stick was identical, black and pretty much the same size.

Feeling rather stupid, I then went through the entire film in silence.

Gone forever.

When I had my previous implant, I had additional batteries. Considering they didn't last as long, I always had a couple with me, to be safe.

I had spent the day in London and I was waiting for the train home, standing a couple of feet away from the platform, looking through the photographs on my camera.

When the power went on my battery, I reached into my pocket awkwardly and pulled the battery out. My hand caught and as I pulled it out, the battery flew from my hand and landed on the floor, narrowly missing going over the edge of the platform.

"Lucky!" I said and went to retrieve it.

At the same time, someone walked past and kicked it, sending it into a crowd of people walking back and forth.

I lost sight of it and started looking around, frustrated, and annoyed.

"What are you doing?" A ticket agent said. "lost something?"

"A battery," I said, removing the second from my pocket to show him. "It's for my implant."

"Implant?" The man said curiously. "What kind of implant?" He almost looked horrified.

"Hearing aid," I said. "Cochlear implant." I took the second battery from my pocket and carefully swapped it.

"I understand," The man said and proceeded to help me look for it, and a couple of minutes later he found it, and unfortunately it had been crushed and was becoming warm.

"Oh dear," I said feeling it getting hotter. "I think this is going to catch alight."

"Hold on," The man said and pulled a bottle of water from his bag, unscrewing the cap and then dropping the battery into the bottle, shaking it.

"That should sort it," He said.

"Thanks," I replied.

"Is it fixable?" He said looking at it inside the bottle.

"No," I said. "That is long dead."

This time, messing around with the battery, I missed my train and had a forty-five-minute wait for the next one. Lucky for me, I managed to get a couple of spare batteries.

Solar Power?

I always meet people who are curious about my implant or my hearing, and sometimes the questions I get are funny, or just plain crazy.

I was at the checkout in a store when the woman behind the counter started a conversation.

> "What is that?" She asked, pointing to my head.
> "It's a cochlear implant," I said. "I am profoundly deaf."
> "Oh," She said. "How does it work?"

I explained briefly how it works, and the operation involved and watched her turn slightly green.

> "That sounds horrible," She said. "Did it hurt?"
> "No," I said. "It was hard psychologically, but I had no pain or anything?"
> "Do you have to change the battery every day?" She asked curiously.
> "Twice a day depending," I said. "I get about nine hours out of a battery on a good day."
> "Do you charge them?" She looked at me. "Or is it solar-powered?"
> "Solar powered?" I said. "Why do you think that?"
> "Isn't that what the black thing on the side of your head is for?" She said.
> "No," I replied. "I have a charging pad at home.

I took the implant off and showed her how the battery comes off, and then put it back on.

> "I thought it was screwed into your head!" She said.
> "No," I replied. "It's a magnet."
> "Sounds horrible," She shivered. "How much can you hear?"
> "About eighty-five percent," I said.
> "So you are not deaf anymore," She smiled. "You must be happy."
> "Still deaf," I said. "Without it, I cannot hear anything."
> "Doesn't seem worth it," She said. "All that cutting and drilling."
> "Well it is very useful when I am wearing it," I replied.
> "If you say so," she said.

I then left, wondering if I could create a solar panel for unlimited power, in the sun obviously.

IPOD

I have an IPOD with a selection of songs on it, something that helps with tinnitus when it gets bad, or when I am writing.

It was half four in the morning and I had just sorted my bag out after a shower, and made myself a coffee and some toast, leaning against the worktop with my eyes closed. That is when I noticed the music, it was loud enough for me to notice, especially after I had turned off the extractor fan.

"Who has music on at this time of the morning," I said to myself. "Bloody loud!"

I walked to the front of the house, looking around in case someone had pulled up with their radio blasting, but couldn't see anyone.

"Sounds like it's in the house," I thought to myself."

It was louder in the hall, so I checked the living room but nothing was on. I then checked the bedrooms, and the study and was even more stumped.

As I came down the stairs, it was louder so I found myself looking through the spyhole and then listening through the letterbox, like the fruitcake I am.

"Where is it coming from?" I said, opening the door and stepping outside. It was a warm summer morning with a gentle breeze. I stood on the doorstep, listening. Trying to work out where it was coming from.

I gave up looking and decided to make my way to work, so I could chill and do some writing before the mad day hit. I cleared up the kitchen, checked everything was turned off and then picked up my rucksack to leave, and then it hit me.

The music got louder at this point and I was thinking, surely the laptop isn't working with the screen closed? I regularly listen to music on YouTube and probably left it on by accident, but there is no chance it ran all night on battery.

I took it out and opened it, silencing it and listening, but the sound wasn't coming from there. I searched through my bag and found the source. My iPod. I hadn't seen it in a while, thinking I had lost it, however, I must have activated it when I was sorting out my bag and it was playing 'Bat out of Hell'.

I felt quite silly at this point and turned it off, leaving it on the stairs and heading to work.

Music on the Bus

Another occasion, probably more embarrassing was a month or so ago when I was on the bus to work. I sat in the middle of the bus, minding my own business and looking out of the window, watching the world go by and wondering what kind of a day I was going to have.

I looked at the seat next to me where a woman sat, and she was eyeballing me.

   "Morning," I said curiously.

She shook her head and huffed, looking away.

I could hear music and it was annoying me, I looked around trying to see where it was coming from.

I don't get people who cannot use headphones or pods, why share the music with everyone, especially when half of the bus is snoring away?

Again the woman opposite me was glaring at me.

   "What's up?" I asked her.
   "Do you have to have that so loud?" She asked.
   "It's not me," I said and looked behind me at a middle-aged man who slowly nodded.
   "It is," He said.

I took out my mobile and checked it, confirming it was off and then checked the laptop, which was also off. I put my ear to the bag, noticing it was louder and then remembered the IPOD.

"Bloody thing," I said. "How does it turn itself on?!"

I rummaged around until I found it and then turned it off.

"Sorry about that," I said in embarrassment. "Couldn't hear it, I am profoundly deaf."
"Why do you have an IPOD if you are deaf?" The woman asked.
"I can still hear it," I replied. "If it's connected to my implant."
"Weird," She said. "Didn't think a deaf person could hear music."
"Oh we can," I said. "Sorry to disturb you."
"It's annoying," She said.
"Give the guy a break," The man behind me said. "He said sorry, what more do you want?"

The woman then moved to the front of the bus, giving me some evil looks as she sat down.

Probably didn't like the options I had…

Since that incident, I now turn it off.

JOURNEY TO CORNWALL

With my car out of action, I decided to take a train to Cornwall for a long weekend to visit friends. Stupidly enough, I expected the journey to be problem-free, something it was far from.

Everything went fine until I got to Paddington to take a train to Plymouth and got on the heavily packed train, hoping my reserved seat was available, or a few hours of standing.

I got to my seat and a young woman was sitting in my seat, her bags in the other.

"That is my seat," I said pointing to the window seat.
"Fancy swapping?" She asked.
"Fine by me," I said.

I sat down and got comfortable, constantly moving for everyone who walked past me, bashing me with either their bags or their elbows, it was going to be a long journey.

The woman next to me tapped my shoulder and when I looked around, she started to sign.

"Oh I don't sign," I said. "Sorry."
"Okay," She said. "I was just curious."
"It's fine," I smiled.
"How deaf are you?" She asked, looking at the implant.
"Completely," I said. "The implant gives me about eighty-five percent."
"That is impressive," She said.

An hour into the journey I put my iPod on, connected to my implant Bluetooth and closed my eyes, relaxing.

I felt a tap on my shoulder and turned around, my head coming into contact with a staff member's head. He groaned and stepped back, rubbing his head and I did the same.

"Could you not hear me over that?" He said. "That hurt!"
"Sorry," I said. "Hurt me too, why were you so close?"

"I was going to speak into your ear," He said. "I noticed you are deaf after trying to get your attention, so thought to shout in your ear."

"Glad you didn't," I said. "Wouldn't have gone well, what did you want?"

"Can I see your ticket?" He said. "This gentleman said you are in his seat."

I looked at the man standing behind him, dressed in a dark grey suit looking very put out.

"Sure," I said and handed him the ticket.

"Looks like you are in the right seat," he said. "And you have it for the duration of the journey."

"So where am I sitting?" The man said.

"Come with me," He said. "I will find you somewhere else to sit."

The man looked at me, shaking his head in annoyance.

"Sorry," I said. "Hardly my fault is it?"

There were serious issues on the train with many seats being double booked, and some angry people getting into arguments, in the end, I switched off my hearing aids, just for the peace.

The rest of the journey went well, other than delays of half an hour which messed up connecting trains. This just meant that on the journey from Plymouth to Truro, I was standing.

I ended up standing near the doors, writing notes for a book, (The Undertaker) and trying to pass the time.

A door opened and a kid walked out, looking around until he saw the toilets, he opened the door, saw the mess, and then went into the opposite unit.

Five minutes passed and a woman came out, looking around in concern.

"Have you seen a boy?" She asked.

"Earlier," I said. "I think he used the toilet."

The woman opened the first one, groaning at the mess and smell and then looked at the second door, knocking on it.

"Are you in there?" She said before opening the door to find the boy, tearful.

She looked at me, annoyed.

"He has been calling for help," She said. "The door was stuck, why didn't you help him?"
"I didn't hear anything," I said. "Otherwise I would have."
"Oh rubbish!" She said.
"I didn't," I said again. "I am deaf, over the noise of the train, I can barely hear anything."
"You could have tried!" She scoffed.
"How could I have tried?" I said. "Seriously, grow up and go away."

She stood there complaining, so I reached up and turned off my hearing aids. She eventually left.

Half an hour or so later, a female member of staff came through, standing in front of me to get my attention.

"Tickets please," She said.

I showed her the tickets.

"Are you going to Truro?" She asked.

It was obvious she knew I was deaf, speaking clearly and slowly.

"Yes," I said.
"Do you need any help with anything?" She asked.
"No," I shook my head.
"Good," She smiled. "If you do, then let me know."

Just before arriving at Truro, I was looking out of the window and when I turned around, there was a little old lady standing so close to me, I thought she was trying to kiss me!

"Are you getting off at Truro?" She asked softly.
"Yes," I said.

"Me too," She smiled.

For a minute I thought she may have been confused, or just overly friendly.

"May I ask you something?" She asked.

"Sure," I said.

"Would you be kind enough to carry off the train onto the platform?" She asked.

"Of course," I said. "Not a problem."

I noticed the woman had a hearing aid on one side.

"I have a hearing aid too," She said. "It was very expensive."

"Okay," I said nodding. "Mine too."

The female member of staff I had spoken to earlier came up behind her.

"Is this your mother?" She asked.

"No," I said.

"Do you need help with your luggage?" She said to the woman.

"No," She said. "This man is going to do it for me."

The train arrived at the station and I got off, lifting off the luggage and then placing it down for her.

"Thank you," She said.

And then patted me on the butt, something that took me by surprise as I sat down, waiting for the next train, watching her leave so she didn't try anything like it again…

NOISES IN THE MORGUE

It was a quiet day at the undertakers funnily enough, and I had spent most of the morning building and dressing the coffins for the week ahead.

I was sitting in the tearoom with a cup of coffee when one of the undertakers, Art popped in.

"You good?" He asked.
"Fine," I said. "Anything exciting happening?" I asked curiously, hoping for a collection.
"No," Art said. "It's a quiet day."
"Is there anything that needs doing?" I asked. "Anything?"

It was the pre-mobile phone times, so I couldn't even sit there and scroll through Instagram.

"Let me think," He said. "There is but it's boring," He said.
"I don't mind," I replied. "I am bored!"
"The cold store needs cleaning," He said.

This was perfect as it was hot and stuffy, and the cold room was chilled, I jumped at the offer.

"I'll take it," I said.

I had helped Art clean it a few days before, getting high on the cleaning spray.

"You okay to do it on your own?" He asked.
"Yes," I said. "Keep me busy for an hour or two."
"Good lad," He said. "You know where everything is?"
"Yes," I said. "Do you want the spare trolley cleaned too?"
"Go for it," Art said. "It's in the hall."
"The one with the squeaky wheel?" I laughed.

I found out the first time moving it, that it sounds like a cat holding on to the wheel when moving it, squealing and squeaking like crazy.

I had been in the cold storage for ten minutes, cleaning down the two trollies when I heard someone call out.

"Hello!" A voice said. "It's cold!"

I have always struggled with locating sounds, so I turned around, expecting to see someone in the doorway.

"Someone there?" I said loudly.

I walked into the corridor, looking down towards the main building and then outside towards the loading area.

"Did someone say something?" I asked again.

I returned to the cold store, looking at the line refrigeration unit, and noticing the handprints and stains.

"That needs a good clean," I thought to myself and returned to cleaning the trolley.

I decided to tip the trolley on the side to properly clean the wheels and hopefully kill the annoying squeak.

"Hello!" A voice came again and I suddenly turned around, knocking the trolley.

The trolley flipped over with a loud echoing clang and I flinched, pausing and watching the door.

I heard footsteps and Art appeared at the doorway, chuckling softly.

"What on earth are you doing?" he asked. "I felt that down the corridor!"
"Sorry," I said. "I was cleaning the wheels."
"Well you are dedicated," Art laughed softly. "Didn't hurt yourself did you?"
"No," I replied. "Got distracted by voices."
"Voices?" Art said looking around curiously. "There is no one about, so do you mean the ones in your head kid?"
"Ha bloody ha," I rolled my eyes. "No, I could hear someone saying hello."

"Right," Art said listening. "Well everyone in here is dead," He nodded, well we only have four bodies and trust me, they are very dead."

"Can you lend a hand?" I pointed to the trolley. "It's awkward."

Art helped me turn the trolley onto the wheels, moving it back and forth.

"Looks like you solved the squeak," He said. "Either that or it's just the wet."

"Needs new wheels," I said. "One is worn."

"You can convince the boss!" He scoffed. "She may listen to you!"

The manager appeared at the doorway.

"What was the almighty bang?" She asked. "Anyone hurt?"

"That was my fault," I said. "It slipped."

"He has cured the squeak though," Art said. "Had to put up with that annoying thing for years."

"Brilliant," She said.

"Hello!" the voice called out again.

"What an earth!" The manager yelped. "Get out!"

One of the compartments clicked and opened.

"You silly sod!" Art said.

"I was only playing," Nick laughed.

"Told you I could hear voices," I said. "Wasn't imagining it."

"Dave is deaf," Art said. "Had no idea where it was coming from, you daft plank!"

"It's okay," I said. "Should have locked it."

"Oh charming," Nick said as he pulled him out of the compartment. "I'd have died!"

"Well, "I replied. "At least you were in the right place!"

HEAD BANGING RESTAURANT

I headed to the local shopping centre to get a few bits and then grab dinner at one of the restaurants, I really fancied pasta.

I got the bits I needed and headed to the restaurant only to be distracted by the cinema and tempted to go in and watch a film.

"Another time," I said to myself. "It's been a long day."

I went to the restaurant, hoping they would have a table considering it was busy.

"How many?" The waitress asked.

I looked behind and then back at her.

"Just me," I said. "Unless you are counting my seven other personalities?"

I don't think she was in the mood for jokes, she looked at me, shaking her head slightly.

"I'll leave the seven outside," I said. "Just one."
"Bar or table?" she said.
"Don't mind," I said. "Happy with either."
"One minute, "She smiled and walked off.

I felt a tap on my shoulder and turned around to find someone I used to work with at the hotel. She was one of the general managers, and we had some very interesting times. (You can read all about these in The Night Porter)

"Hi," I said. "How are you?"
"Great," She said. "Long time no see, what are you up to?"
"Grabbing some food," I said. "You?"
"Funny," She rolled her eyes. "Fancy sharing a table?"
"Sure," I said as the waitress came over. "Change of plan, table for two."

The waitress seated us at the table.

"So what are you doing these days?" She asked. "Been years since you walked out of the hotel that night."

"Blimey," I said. "Feels like yesterday. So much has happened," I sighed. "Went into retail after I walked, right up until two thousand and four when I got made redundant."

"You are one unlucky sod," She scoffed. "Then?"

"Took a volunteer role at the hospital," I said. "Then a paid job, now working in medical engineering and supervising."

"Wow," She nodded. "Big change then!"

"Yeah," I said. "been a very busy few years. How about you?"

"I left," she said. "A relative left me a ton of money, so I went travelling around Australia for a couple of years, and then America, when I got back I set up my own company, Wedding planning."

"Oh wow," I nodded. "Sounds interesting, when did you leave the hotel?"

"About three months after you," she said. "I had a very handsy customer and had him thrown out, turns out he was friends with the owner, so they asked me to apologise."

"I guess that went well," I laughed.

"How did the tribunal go?" she asked. "Last I heard was the hotel manager freaking out because you were taking him to a tribunal."

"It was thrown out," I said. "So neither of us won, but when you look at it, they did."

"Toxic place," She scoffed. "Probably did us both good getting out."

The waitress came to the table.

"Do you need more time or…?" She asked.

"I know what I am having," I said. "Do you?"

"Yes," She said. "You go first."

"Could I have the Polo Pesto and a side of garlic bread," I said. "And water please."

"Creepy," She said. "I will have the same."

The waitress smiled and left, walking back to the counter.

"That is the only reason I come here," She said. "That is my favourite dish."

"Me too," I said. "Do you live local?"

"Bromley," She said. "You?"

"Longfield," I said. "Not too far."

"Married? Children?" She asked curiously.

"No," I said. "There is someone I really like but she isn't interested."

"There is someone out there," She smiled. "No children for me, but I am married."

"That is amazing," I said. "Happy for you, how did you meet him?"

"Her," She said. "We met in an airport in America after our internal flight was cancelled, she wasn't too well so I kept an eye on her."

"Everything happens for a reason huh?" I said.

"Turns out she also lived local to me," She said. "So we met up, didn't expect anything other than friendship, to be honest, I wasn't sure myself."

"Went well obviously," I said. "Who proposed?"

"She did," She chuckled. "In Las Vegas!"

"No!" I groaned. "Whereabouts?"

"Well we went to see a show, Fantasy I think it was," She said.

"Seen it," I replied. "About three times."

"Great minds," she winked. "We then went to Freemont to try out the burger place," she sat there thinking," Heart attack grill or something."

"No," I said. "She didn't propose there?!"

"No," She laughed. "She proposed in front of a live band, they were doing a cover of, We Will Rock You!"

"Love that," I said. "First song I heard when I went there. When was this?"

"Two years ago," She said. "We are currently looking at adoption now."

"Kids?" I asked.

"Behave!" She groaned. "Dogs."

"Right answer," I said.

The waitress came over with the water and garlic bread, placing it on the table.

"When did you go to Vegas?" She asked.

"Last year," I said. "Going again for New Year."

"Who with?" She asked curiously.

"Just me," I said. "Christmas in Yosemite, Zion, Grand Canyon and then Vegas."

"Very nice," She nodded.

Her phone went off and she picked it up, checking it.

"Sorry I need to grab this," she nodded, standing up and walking to the doors.

A minute passed and leaned back slightly to stretch my back and felt a dull thud against my head, followed by ice-cold liquid going down my back and I stood up in fright. My shoulder came in contact with a waitress carrying our pasta, sliding off the tray onto the table next to us.

Following the crashing of glass and crockery, all eyes were on me.

"Did you not hear me say excuse me?" The waitress said.
"No," I said. "I didn't," I was pulling at the wet cold shirt sticking to my back.
"Why not," She said in annoyance. "Are you deaf?"
"Yes," I nodded. "Completely," I pointed to my hearing aids.

Eyes were then on the waitress.

"What happened?" A supervisor came to the table. "Are you okay?"
"Fine," I said. "It was an accident."
"Could you get some help," He said to the waitress. "Let's get these tables sorted and some fresh meals."
"What happened Dave?" my friend said. "Did you try to have the food all to yourself?"

I explained what had happened and she covered her mouth, laughing.

Lucky for me, I had a T-shirt in my bag so I went and got changed, by the time I came back, they had cleaned the tables and sorted out the food which was on the house.

We then walked around the shopping centre for a while as she wanted my advice on some books, so I recommended a few by Stephen King.

The wet trousers didn't make the evening or the drive home much fun.1166

ORDER

I took a day off to get a replacement microwave after mine had failed after a couple of weeks, leaving the house stinking of electrical burning for several months.

Following the delivery map, I could see when the driver was nearby and it was due at midday. I had planned to head out for lunch and do some shopping, however the courier had other plans.

I had a couple of missed calls on my phone but ignored them as I didn't recognise the numbers. I searched for them, however nothing came up.

Seeing the van was at the end of the street, I stood by the window, waiting. I had the fault one boxed up and ready for him to collect.

I watched as the van drove down, and even stopped outside my house, delivering to the house opposite, however had nothing for me and I watched him get in the van and drive away.

My phone beeped and I had a message stating the driver had been delayed, which I thought was curious considering he was right outside my house.

The doorbell buzzed about an hour later followed by loud knocking. I could barely hear it over the sound of the television.

"Great," I said and opened the door, to find a courier standing there with a small parcel.
"You deaf or something mate?" He said. "Been ringing your doorbell."
"Profoundly," I said pointing to my hearing aids. "Didn't hear the door."
"Sorry," He said. "Can you take this for next door?"
"I suppose so," I said.
"They aren't answering," He said. "And I don't want to come back."
"Don't suppose you have anything for me?" I asked.
"No," He said.

I waited all day, and he finally turned up at seven in the evening, casually walking up to the door and dropping the parcel down on the step as I opened it.

"How come this wasn't delivered at lunchtime?" I asked. "You were practically outside my house."

"It was busy," he said. "I called you this morning and you agreed to change the times."

"No one has called me," I said.

"Well I spoke to you," He said. "Can you just confirm your name please?"

"You didn't speak to me," I added. "I cannot even hear on the phone."

"Why not?" He asked.

"I am deaf," I said.

The look on his face was brilliant, even when he was struggling to find his words.

"Maybe I spoke to someone else?" He said.

"No," I said. "No one here but me."

"Well it is here now," He said. "What is the problem?"

"Just don't understand why you were outside my house at lunchtime and the map said I was next," I said. "I wasted a whole day sitting around waiting."

"Well I cannot control deliveries," He said. "And I went to get dinner, so the map changes depending on where I am."

"I hope it isn't broken after you dropped it like a sack of potatoes," I said.

"You like to complain don't you?" He scoffed.

"I have a parcel for collection," I said.

"I am not collecting anything," He said.

"It's on the delivery," I added. "If you don't take it, they will charge me for the new one."

"Not my problem," He said. "Take it up with the seller."

He then stormed off.

Lucky for me I didn't have to pay for the new unit, and it appears several people had complained that day about the courier and his attitude.

Was annoying having to get rid of a blown-up microwave that stunk out the house.

RAKE!

There were times I struggled to understand my aunt to the point we were both in hysterics. One weekend, my grandmother came over for dinner and I was doing odds and ends around the house, while my aunt and grandmother sorted out the dinner.

I was up in the loft, clearing out the many books I had after a leak destroyed most of them, it was a frustrating and sad day.

"David?" My grandmother called out. "Are you in your room?"

"No, I am up here!" I said.

"Heaven?" She laughed.

"No, the loft you Wally!" I looked down from the loft as she appeared at the top of the stairs.

"Margaret said could you pop to the shop and get some cream?" She rolled her eyes. "For the trifle."

"I got that yesterday," I said. "Surely that isn't all gone?"

"I'll look in the fridge," She laughed.

My aunt had a habit of forgetting what she had, someone who always had at least five loaves of bread in the house, but still wanted me to pop out and get one just in case she had to feed the five thousand.

I came down after twenty minutes and sat by the window with a drink, watching my aunt and grandmother in the garden, pulling weeds.

I knocked on the window to get their attention.

"Missed a bit!" I said and laughed.

My aunt looked at me and said, overemphasising her words.

"No dinner for you!" She poked her tongue out.

My aunt always struggled with how lip-reading worked and because she forced it so much behind windows, I struggled with understanding her.

She said something and I asked her to repeat it, but to me, it sounded like 'Can you put the weed on." So I went out to speak to her.

"Can I put the weed on?" I said. "You have weed?"

My grandmother burst into hysterics along with my aunt who was now unable to talk properly with the giggles.

"Are you some kind of drug dealer or something?!" I said in mock shock.
"What are you talking about?" She said. "How old are you?"
"Physical age or mental age?" I asked.

My grandmother was laughing, shaking her head.

"You are mental," My aunt rolled her eyes. "I give you that."
"Charming," I scoffed. "No dessert for you."
"Well there is no point in me making it then," She said poking her tongue out.
"I'll make it for him," My grandmother said. "He is taking me home!"
"Ah at least someone loves me," I said defiantly. "What did you say?"
"I said could you put the greens on," My aunt said.
"Bloody hell," I snapped. "Weed sounds better."

I went into the kitchen and sorted out the vegetables, putting the hobs on and waiting for the water to boil. A few minutes later my grandmother walked in.

"I'll do that," She said. "Marg wants your help."

I went out into the garden, walking up to the flower beds where she was weeding.

"You called?" I said.
"Can you move those bricks?" She said pointing to the dozen or so bricks by the gate.
"Where to?" I asked.
"Down the side of the storage cupboard," She pointed to the large plastic mini shed by the window.
"Sure," I nodded.

I moved the bricks, piling them up against the wall.

"Where is the broom?" I asked.
"Why?" She said. "Are you going for a fly?"
"No," I nodded. "I prefer driving, I will leave the flying to you."
"Cheeky bugger!" She glared at me. "It's in the cupboard, why do you need it?"
"Have a wild guess," I replied sarcastically.
"You are going the right way for a smack," She pointed at me in warning. "I'll do it, can you pull up this weed, it's tough."

I went to pull the weed out, misjudging how tough it was and nearly pulled myself into the flower bush, watching my grandmother laughing in the window.

"Dave!" My aunt yelled out. "Rake!"
"Rake?" I said curiously. "Didn't know you had a rake."
"Dave!" She screamed, frozen on the spot.

My grandmother was looking through the window curiously and concerned.

"What?" I walked over calmly.

As I approached her, she yelped and turned, dropping the broom and shoving me. I stepped back, tripping over a large plant pot on the edge of the patio and fell heavily onto the grass, banging my head and seeing a mass of stars.

My aunt ran into the house, slamming the patio door behind her and locking it.

I sat up, looking at my grandmother in the window in hysterics.

"What the hell just happened?" I asked her through the window.
She shrugged her shoulders, unable to speak through laughter.

I got up and went to open the patio door, only to find it locked. I knocked and my grandmother came to it, trying to open it.

"It's jammed!" She said. "I cannot unlock it."

"I'll go round to the front," I said. "Has she gone nuts?"

I walked round to the front of the house and rang the doorbell, waiting a minute until my aunt opened it, looking rather worried.

"What was that about?" I asked. "What's with the rake?"

"It was a snake you Wally," She said.

Lipreading my aunt was a struggle when she was in a panic.

"Oh that makes more sense," I replied.

"Did you hurt yourself?" She asked.

"No," I replied. "You did that when you shoved me and left me at the mercy of the snake!" I rolled my eyes, hearing my grandmother giggle from the kitchen. My aunt had a fear of rats, mice and snakes.

While they sorted dinner, I unjammed the patio door and went outside into the garden to investigate the snake. Only to find a small plastic-coated metal hook by the wall, it originally was red, but was now a pale pink from the years of sun damage.

I picked it up and looked at them both through the window, panic on my aunt's face and my grandmother looked closer and then burst into fits of hysterics. I put it into the bin and went back into the house, shaking my head.

"What was it?" She asked.

"A hook," I said. "Remember the two holding the ladder on under the window seal?"

"Oh!" She exclaimed.

"We took the ladder down because she kept hearing the rain tapping against it in the middle of the night," I said. "Drove her nuts."

"Didn't it bother you?" My aunt said.

"Have a wild guess," I glared at her.

My grandmother continued to laugh, so much she was crying.

ROGER

I have a Bluetooth receiver that connects to both my implant and hearing aid, brilliant for listening to music on my iPod and also for team meetings at work, it is a small device that easily fits in a pocket, so it doesn't take up much room.

No doubt you are wondering where Roger comes into this story, but it isn't as exciting as you think. Roger is the name of the receiver. My implant is called the Marvel, so when I explain this to people, it always generates a giggle when Roger comes up.

I get to work early every day, to get some writing done before I start and I always aim for at least two thousand words a day. It was a Monday and I decided to pop into the local coffee shop and get some food and a strong coffee. I didn't sleep well and had been up since midnight, so I needed a very strong coffee.

"Good morning," The barista said. "How can I help you?"
"Could I have a cappuccino please," I said handing the two bacon rolls to her. "And these please."
"Take away?" She asked.
"Yes please," I said.
"What size?" She said.
"Medium will be fine," I smiled. "One plate for those too."
"Hungry?" She asked.
"Yes," I said. "And greedy!"

She laughed and prepared them while I found a table in the corner, removing my laptop and iPod.

A few minutes later, she called me over so I collected the drink and food and sat down to eat.

The noise in the coffee shop was overwhelming, with the air con unit humming and the coffee machines constantly making some noise.

"Time for some music," I said, and plugged Roger into the iPod, turning it on.

I selected the soundtrack for the Rocky Horror Picture Show, the stage version, and started it while I did some writing.

Every time someone came into the coffee shop, they looked towards me, either smiling or nodding, or a general good morning.

I was there for just over an hour and the album had finished and moved on to the next one.

The barista came over, standing at the end of the table and smiling.

"Hello," She said. "My colleague and I wanted to thank you for the music."
"Music?" I said curiously.

And then it hit me.

"You could hear that?" I asked. "Really?"
"I am a regular Frankie fan," She said. "Love Rocky horror!"

Imagine my horror when I realised that it was blasting out from the corner of the coffee shop for all to hear.

"I am so sorry," I said. "I am not entirely sure how the bloody thing works."

I have no idea why, but sometimes it switches from direct to my implant to, implant and speaker.

"Don't be," She said. "It made our morning."
"Didn't anyone complain?" I asked, packing away my things.
"No," She said. "We had a couple of people ask if it could be turned up."

The other barista came over to the table, putting a cappuccino to go.

"On the house," She said. "Don't dream it," She smiled.
"Well I am glad everyone enjoyed it," I stood up. "Thanks for the coffee."
"Have you seen it live?" The first barista asked.
"Three times," I said. "Loved it."

98

"Five times for me," She said. "What did you think of the remake?"

"It was okay," I said. "but didn't have a soul like the original."

"I agree," She said.

"I had better go," I said. "Thanks for everything."

I made my way to work, wondering if it had happened before.

The only time it did was when I was in a team's meeting, and my colleagues could hear everything being said.

ROUGE GOLF BALL

It was early in the morning, and I had just finished work, dropped off a friend and then was heading home, popping into my aunts on the way.

Tired, hungry and warm. I rolled down the window for some fresh air and a distraction from the tiredness.

I was only a few minutes from my aunt's house, passing a golf course on the way and I slowed down as the traffic started to build up from people pulling into the golf course car park.

"Come on!" I moaned at the cars that had blocked the road, rather than use the right lane for turning into the course. Eventually, a car moved, creating space and I sped up, glancing at the large golf course as I went past.

Something hit me on the side of the head on the temple, sharp pain and stars exploded. I briefly lost control, grabbing the wheel and straightening up when a car in the opposite direction flashed me. I pulled onto the grass verge, fighting the urge to throw up, my head spinning.

I sat there for a few minutes, distracted by someone looking into the car.

"I am really sorry," The man said. "It's my fault, are you okay?"
"What happened?" I asked, looking around, struggling to focus. "What the hell hit me?"

I thought it had been a bird or something, my hand going up to the side of my head, expecting blood.

"My golf ball," The man said. "I hit it too hard, in the wrong direction!"
"Golf ball?!" I scoffed, the pain getting worse. "Jesus Christ!" I moaned.

He called an ambulance after I got out of the car, struggling to focus and walk straight, I fell backwards into the grass and fought to stay conscious, only to slowly pass out with the thick grass around me.

I woke a few minutes later, looking up at the man and a police officer. They were both talking to me, but I couldn't understand, the light blinding me.

"I cannot understand," I said. "I am deaf."

"Oh no, what have I done!" The man panicked as the officer helped me sit up.

"I was deaf before," I said. "Nothing to do with you."

"Are you okay?" The officer asked, bending down and looking at me closely. "The side of your head is swelling."

"A golf ball to the face would do that," I tried to joke. "I feel sick!"

An ambulance arrived sometime later, a female paramedic kneeling next to me, checking over me, taking my blood pressure and checking my else, the lump on the side of my head growing.

"We will need to take you in," She said. "The fact you feel sick isn't good."

"Is there anything I can do?" The man said. "I feel so bad."

"Do you live nearby?" The officer asked.

"About five minutes," I replied.

"Let me put his car in the carpark," The man said. "I will let them know what has happened."

"Are you okay with that?" The officer said looking at me.

"Sure," I nodded and groaned. "That is okay, keys are still in the car."

They walked me to the ambulance, monitoring me and giving me oxygen when I started to feel dizzy and sick again.

I had an x-ray, did the usual checks with the consultant and was given pain relief. The lump on my head made me look like a post-apocalyptic freak, the swelling and bruising making it hard for me to fully open my eyes. The consultant was sure my eye socket was fractured, pointing out minor damage which was from when I had my corrective eye surgery as a toddler. He seemed pretty frustrated when I corrected him.

A nurse also caused some worry when she called an audiologist to check my hearing, when she failed to read my notes that pointed out my severe hearing loss was not a result of the golfing shot.

I fell asleep, only to be woken a short while later by the man who had achieved the impressive shot through my window, nearly replacing my useless left eye with a golf ball.

"How are you feeling?" He asked. "I am really sorry mate."

"It was an accident," I said. "Impressive shot though!" I laughed.

"Here," He said handing me an envelope.

"What is it?" I asked. "A summons for the damaged ball?"

He laughed and shook his head.

"No," He said. "It's an apology."

I opened the envelope and found it full of cash.

"Woah," I said in shock. "What's this for?"

"Anything you want," The man said. "It's my way of saying sorry."

"You don't have to do this," I said. "It was an accident."

"It's okay," The man said. "If you need anything, just let me know. This is my email address and phone number."

He handed me a small business card.

"Thanks," I said.

I felt awful taking the money, but considering he was a solicitor, I doubt he would have missed it.

"When are they letting you out?" He asked.

"Soon," I replied. "They wanted to keep me in overnight, but no chance."

I hated hospitals, and definitely not staying for the night.

He stayed with me and then dropped me home, explaining that he told the golf course why my car was there and that he would pay for the parking if needed. He gave me the keys back and I went straight to bed, falling asleep instantly.

I woke up the next morning and the pain was mental, the image in the mirror no better with the unsightly lump on the side of my head and the minor black eye.

I didn't go to work, emailing and explaining the situation and I went back to bed. Sleeping much of the day, waking when I needed to drink and complain about the throbbing headache.

I picked up the car the next day, on the way to work.

The story generated some giggles and gasps at work, and certainly some sympathy for the mini-head that had occupied the side of my head for a few days.

It was a month or so until the tenderness disappeared, and I avoided the golf course. Where I couldn't, the window was wound up.

A few days later, a golf ball was posted through my letter box with a smiley face drawn on it. I no longer have it after walloping it into the sea at Gravesend Beach many years ago, however, I wonder if it was the one that tried to kill me?

SIGNING KID

I was sat in a waiting room at the implant team in London, waiting for my appointment for a hearing test and check-up.

A woman sat opposite me with her young daughter, who waved at me as she sat down.

"Hi," The woman said. "Is that new?" She pointed at my implant.

"Yes," I said. "Got it last year."

"How are you finding it?" She asked curiously.

"Brilliant," I said. "Do you have one?"

"No," She said. "My daughter is going to have surgery soon for two."

"Oh wow," I said. "That is great. How old is she?"

"Five," She said. "And drives me up the wall."

The girl started to sign to her mother, looking at me with shyness.

"She asked if you were deaf," The woman said and signed back.

"Oh cool," I nodded.

"She asked if you know sign language?" She asked.

"No," I said. "Never learnt and wasn't encouraged or given the opportunity."

She signed to her daughter, explaining what I had said. The girl rolled her eyes as she signed and the mother laughed.

"What?" I asked. "What did she say."

"She said what stopped you learning now you are grown up?" She laughed.

"That is a very good point," I said.

The girl faced me and signed slowly.

"What is she saying?" I asked.

"She said that sign language is so much fun," The woman said. "And that, strangely, you cannot sign."

She tapped on the girl's shoulder and spoke as she signed.

"Not all deaf people sign," She said.

The girl looked at me and signed to her mother.

"Were you born deaf?" She asked.
"No," I replied. "I went deaf at seven."
"How?" She asked.
"Dodgy genetics," I said.

The mother explained it to her daughter.

"Can you hear much with your implant?" She asked.
"So much," I said. "It has been amazing."
"She said she is getting two," The mother laughed. "Wanted to rub that in your face."
"Fair enough," I laughed.
"She also said it's easier to talk in private when you can sign," The mother said and shoved her daughter gently. "Is that what you and nanny do?"

The girl nodded and giggled.

I always wanted to learn to sign and still do, one of those things I can never seem to dedicate myself to.

STICKS AND STONES

Being deaf and wearing glasses, I was a target of the bullies at mainstream school. I was short and skinny, nervous and timid. I wasn't fast on my feet, so running away never worked to my advantage.

Students were the worst bullies, but believe me, so were teachers.

Sports

There was a time at primary school when I forgot my sports gear and it was football, so I decided to sit out in the changing rooms and read.

It was a half-hour into the session and I got up to look out of the window, to see what was going on.

I didn't hear the teacher come up behind me, she was in charge of the deaf unit at the school where there were a small number of deaf students, and she would provide support (if you call it that). I didn't hear her, but I felt what followed.

She slapped me across the backside, so hard I lost my balance and my head hit the window. The stinging pain was unbearable. I shot round to find the teacher looking down at me, anger on her face.

  "Why are you not in sports?" She demanded.
  "Forgot my kit," I said, my voice trembling.
  "Then you should have told the teacher," She said. "We would have got something from lost property!"
  "Sorry," I said quietly.
  "Hold out your hand!" She said.

I reluctantly held out my hand.

  "Do as you're told," She brought her hand down, cracking me across the top of my hand. "Go to my office!" She snapped.

My hand was bruised the next day and I had to put up with her crap for some time, she wasn't any fun at all. There was another incident where again, sports events, something I was never good at or enjoyed. I found myself exploring spider webs on the local bushes, my back turned to the games.

"David!" She yelped, slapping me across the backside so hard, that I fell to the floor, dazed. She then yanked me up by the arm, shoving me towards the field. "Don't let me catch you slacking again!"

All eyes were on me as I limped back to the field.

When I went to secondary school, I was bullied all the time.

School Bullies

It was a normal lunchtime at secondary school, hanging around in the fields with friends and eating our food. My friends went to play football, something I hated with a passion, and did my best to avoid.

I was sitting on a railing, finishing my sandwich and about to open a coke, when this boy from a couple of years above me walked over.

"Can I have that?" He asked, pointing to the coke.
"It's mine," I said.
"I want it," He held out his hand. "Hand it over."
"No," I said and moved the coke closer to me.

He kicked out, hitting me in the chest and sending me back over the railings. I landed heavily on the floor, knocking the air out of me and seeing a mass of stars.

"Retard," He scoffed, picking up the coke and eyeballing me as he downed it in one go, letting out a belch and then throwing the can at me.

It bounced off my face with a clunk.

"Bully," I said and stood up. "Why don't you pick on someone your own size."
"Got any food?" He asked with a grin.
"No," I said and glanced at my bag as I stood up.

He grabbed the bag, looked through it and pulled out an apple and banana.

"You some kind of mummies boy?" He scoffed and threw the apple at me, hitting me in the face.
"Leave me alone," I said.
"What is this," He pulled out the pouch that had my radio microphone and loop.
"Careful," I said. "That is expensive."

He dropped it to the floor and kicked it.

"Oops!" He said in sarcasm.

He peeled the banana and ate it greedily.

"Pig," I mumbled.
"What you say?" He asked me.
"You are a bully and a pig!" I said.

He ran at me, grabbing me and dragging me over the railings and I tried to fight him off, but he was too big. One of my friends came over.

"Sticks and stones!" I yelled at him.
"Pathetic," He snapped. "This is going to be fun!"
"Come on," He said. "Leave him alone, he is deaf."
"Why should I care?" The bully said, getting me into a headlock.
"You are going to break his heading aids," My friend said. "Come on man."
"You want to go next?" He warned him.
"No," He said. "Let him go, you already took his stuff."
"Let me go!" I started to panic, I had a thing about being restricted. "Let me go please!" I begged him.

The bully held tightly on my neck and then fell backwards, smashing my head into the soft dirt, sending a mass of stars in my eyes. He then got up, kicking me between the legs and I yelped, curling up into a foetal position, sobbing quietly as he walked away. I started to taste blood, and my nose also bleeding.

108

"You okay?" My friend asked.
"Leave me alone," I cried.

I lay in the dirt for some time, and the teachers were far from sympathetic when I showed up for class with muddy trousers.

Lockers

The next year was no different, even though it would be my last year at mainstream school before going to a boarding school for the deaf, it was still hard.

There was one guy, that seemed to enjoy bullying me, also responsible for throwing my hearing aids and glasses off the bridge that connected both school sites.

It was winter and freezing. I got a hot drink, an orange MaxPax from the vending machines, disgusting at the best of times, but refreshing. I sat out the back, in the slight drizzle to hide from this guy, who I knew would be looking for me. It was a courtyard, temporarily set up as a locker dumping ground, with over two hundred single lockers.

My friends and I were messing around the week before, hiding in them and jumping out on each other, I rarely won, due to not being able to hear anyone coming.

"Hiding from me?" The bully said from between the lockers.
"No," I lied.
"What is that?" He asked, pointing to the drink.
"Orange," I said.
"I'll give you a pound for it," He said.

I had paid forty pence for it, so I wasn't going to argue.

"Okay," I said and handed him the drink as he fumbled around in his pocket for the money, dropping fifty pence on the floor.
"Grab that for me," He said.

I bent down to pick it up, and he then poured the piping hot drink over my backside, resulting in me yelling and crying in pain.

"Baby," He said. "Not even that hot."

It burnt like hell, he also caught my lower back.

"Give me my money back," He said. "You made me spill it."
"Oh come on!" I moaned.
"I'll punch your head in!" He warned me.

I handed the money back to him, tears welling up in my eyes from the pain.

"Come here a minute," He said and grabbed me, leading me towards a locker. "Can you fit in here?"
"Yes," I said stupidly enough.
"Get in," He demanded.
"I need to get to class," I said. "Let me go please, I will buy you a drink."
"You gay or something?" He said.
"No," I said.
"Get in!" He snapped.

I got into the locker reluctantly, my back against it as my heart pounded.

"Now what?" I said.
"Stay all night if you want," He said and slammed the door shut, locking it.

He then tipped the locker, and it fell forward, smashing my face into the steel door.

That was when the claustrophobia kicked in, restricted, I went into panic mode.

"Let me out!" I cried. "Please!"

Half an hour passed until someone heard me and tipped the locker back up, finding me with a bloodied nose and face.

110

I was summoned to the headmaster's office and disciplined for messing around in the lockers. Even after explaining what had happened, they refused to believe me because of getting caught by maintenance the week before, messing around.

Being bullied at school became a normal thing for me, and with glasses and hearing aids, I was a target.

<u>Hearing aid</u>

One afternoon before the final lesson of the day, I was tripped on the bridge and one of my hearing aids grabbed from my ear.

I frantically searched everywhere for it but failed to find it, so I made my way to audiology where they had spares.

"What is the matter?" She said as I walked into the room.
"I got tripped on the bridge and someone grabbed my hearing aid," I said tearfully.
"What happened?" She asked.
"I told you," I said.
"What really happened?" She said in annoyance. "You said this happened to you before, so surely you must be careless with your hearing aids."
"Someone tripped me and took it from me," I said. "I looked everywhere."
"Sit down," She said.

I sat down while she went through a drawer.

"You keep losing your equipment," She said. "Do you have any idea how expensive it is?"
"It was taken from me," I said.
"There are children in other countries that don't get things like this," she said. "Do you ever think about them?"

It was pointless arguing, teachers rarely had sympathy for victims.

STREET INTERVIEWER

Popped into town to go to the bank to sort out a couple of issues and pay in some money.

As I left to make my way back to the car a guy started walking towards me with a clipboard, and I was in a rush to try and avoid him.

"Could I have a few minutes," He said.
"Sorry," I said. "I am in a rush," I said holding up my hand.
"I promise I will be quick," He said. "You can have a doughnut."

The option of a doughnut changed everything.

"Okay," I said. "Twist my arm!"

I followed him to the table.

"This is a discussion about headphones," He said showing me a booklet. "Do you use headphones?"
"No," I said. "I am deaf."

He laughed and nodded.

"That is funny," He said.
"Why?" I asked.
"You are not deaf," He added.
"I am," I said. "Profoundly."

He looked up in confusion.

"Completely deaf," I said. "Both ears."
"You cannot be," He exclaimed. "You heard me earlier."
"You came at me like a vulture," I said smiling. "I had no choice".
"Am I that bad?" He scoffed. "So do you?"
"Do I what?" I asked.

"Use headphones?" He said, not looking up from the clipboard.

"No," I said. "I am deaf."

He then looked up, looking at my implant processor.

"Oh, you weren't kidding!" He said.

"No," I said. "I am completely deaf."

"But," He hesitated. "You don't seem it."

"Good at hiding it," I laughed. "My implant gives me about eighty percent and I rely on lip-reading to communicate."

"Lip-reading?" He said putting his clipboard down and handing me a single donut in a small box.

"I read lip patterns," I said.

The man looked at me as if I were making it up.

"That is weird," he said. "Do you have any other superpowers?"

"I am deaf," I said. *"I wasn't bitten by a radioactive spider."*

He laughed.

"It's amazing," He said. "I have never met a deaf person before," He exclaimed. "Wow!"

"You want an autograph?" I said opening the doughnut box. "They cost a doughnut each."

"Hey, Cath!" He called out to a woman at the end of the bench on her phone. "This guy is deaf!"

"Came down," I said. "I am not a circus attraction, don't want people getting jealous."

Cath walked over, looking very uninterested.

"What?" she said.

"Funny," The man laughed.

"No I didn't hear you," She said. "I am deaf in one ear."

The man looked at her and then back at me, and then awkwardly at her again.

"Are you?" He asked.

"Yes," She said. "Told you that this side isn't so good, clearly fell on deaf ears."

113

"Oh wow," He chuckled. "Two deaf people in one day, what are the chances?"

"One in seven," I said, Cath nodded in agreement.

"Do you know each other?" He asked.

"Why?" She said.

"Well you are both deaf," He said. "So I wondered."

"No," I said. "Never met Cath in my life!"

Cath looked at me and grinned, lip-reading a message to me.

"Actually," Cath said. "I think I know you."

"I agree," I said. "I think you are my long-lost twin!" I exclaimed.

She came up to me and hugged me, nearly crushing my doughnut.

"Oh wow!" The man said and then paused. "Are you both winding me up?"

"Of course we are!" She scoffed. "You are an idiot!"

"Sorry," He said. "Anyhow," He looked at the clipboard. "Do you use headphones?"

Cath gave me a pack of four doughnuts and I left, walking away as fast as I could.

The doughnuts were tasty.

STUPIDITY

I usually go shopping without my hearing aids on, due to issues in the past and the fact that the noise is overwhelming. Most of my shopping is done online, but at times like this, I stop at a local just for a few odds and ends. I went in without hearing aids on, but bumped into someone who works at the same trust, so telling them to hold on, I then put my hearing aid back in.

"Hi," I said.

"Hi Dave," She smiled. "Do you not wear your hearing aids?"

"Not usually," I said. "Too noisy."

"Are you at work tomorrow?" She asked.

"No I am not," I said. "Don't work weekends."

"Our monitor is broken," She said. "Can you come in and have a look?"

"No," I said. "You can try the library or ask other wards but it will have to wait until Monday."

"That is a shame," She said. "Do you not work on call?"

"No," I replied.

"Don't suppose you could pop in before you go home?" She said, nearly begging.

"No," I laughed. "I need to go home and chill, it's been a long day," I sighed in annoyance. "What is wrong with it?"

"It won't turn on," She said.

"Is it plugged in?" I asked.

"No we have lost the lead," She said.

"Probably the reason why it won't turn on then," I groaned. "You have a tray in the storeroom full of leads, plug one in and you will find it will work okay."

"I will try that," She said. "Have a nice evening, be careful, you may not hear people talking to you."

"That was the general idea," I said, waving as she walked away.

It had been a long day and I was queuing in a long line at the supermarket, my own fault for avoiding the self-service tills, mainly because I hate them with a passion and they ALWAYS go wrong on me.

It was a Friday evening, fancied something different so I had beers, chicken, korma, rice and naan bread. As well as a few other odds and ends for the weekend. Not forgetting the family trifle, however all for me, I don't share. Not unless you are someone special, then I may share.

Someone tapped on my shoulder when I was third in line, watching the till operator move so slowly, that I even thought time had stopped. I turned around to find a large women, so close to me that she practically stood on my shoes.

"I was talking to you," She said.
"Okay," I replied. "How can I help?"
"Can I push in?" She asked.

I looked at her trolley, nearly full.

"No," I said. "I only have a few items."
"I am in a rush," She said, trying to make me feel sorry for her with her puppy eyes, but she looked more like a rabid bulldog.
"Me too," I said.

I turned around and continued watching the man, struggling to scan a loaf of bread.

The woman tapped me on the shoulder.

"Yes?" I said sighing as I turned and looked at her.
"What is that on your head?" She pointed at the implant processor.
"It's a cochlear implant," I replied.
"What for?" She asked.
"I am deaf," I replied. "Helps me to hear."
"You are deaf?" She said. "So that is why you were ignoring me earlier."
"Well not really ignoring you," I replied. "As I said, deaf."
"Are you sure?" She said.
"Sure of what?" I asked.
"That you are deaf?" She said.
"Yes," I replied. "Have been most of my life and had tons of tests that prove otherwise."
"But you don't look deaf," She laughed.
"That is okay," I said. "You don't look stupid, so we are even."

116

I turned around, grinning. I am pretty sure the man in front of me heard because I could see him laughing when he turned around briefly.

I could hear her behind me, complaining and ranting and just ignored it.

A short while later when the operator was serving me, an employee made her way to the till, waving to get my attention.

"Hello," She said. "We received a complaint that you abused a customer."

I turned around to look at the woman, only to find she had gone.

"Really?" I said. "Absolute rubbish."
"She said you called her stupid," she said. "And said you were very nasty to her."

I looked towards customer service and noticed the woman looking down, with a smile on her face like she had just won a fish at the fair.

"Actually that is incorrect," I said. "I said she didn't look stupid."
"What prompted that?" She asked.
"She said I didn't look deaf," I said shrugging my shoulders. "Could you explain how someone looks deaf?"
"No," She said looking at customer service. "I have a deaf nephew so that is a pretty stupid remark."
"So you get why I said what I did?" I asked, packing my items away at the same time.
"I will send her on her way," She said. "Sorry to bother you."

After I packed and paid, I made my way back to the car, slowing at the customer service and said, slowly and sarcastically.

"This is how we say goodbye in deaf," and gave her a two-fingered salute.

I get some stupid comments from people, but the wannabe queue jumper was a classic.

"You don't look deaf(!)"

TAPS

I rarely wear hearing aids around the house due to tinnitus and also because I love the quiet. There are times when it becomes problematic, however not so sure this is my hearing issue, or more a distraction issue.

I was spring cleaning the house and took my hearing aid before hovering, and that is when the problem started. I had been hoovering the hall, and then the living room but failed to realise that the plug had disconnected from the socket, and I have no idea how long I was hoovering for, wondering why the new hoover was not picking up anything. It was only when I realised that the hoover wasn't sucking, and also not on. So I plugged it back in and then properly ran it around the living room.

A short while later I cleared the kitchen, running the hot tap for a while due to the fact it takes time to heat up, and while I did this, I went into the living room to grab my phone.

I was distracted by an email and grabbed my laptop to look at it in more detail, also putting on the television.

Ten minutes later, I went back to the kitchen to get a drink and froze at the site that welcomed me. Long story short, a bottle of washing-up liquid somehow fell into the washing-up bowl, with hot water gushing into it. The foam had now poured down the side of the cabinet and covered half of the kitchen floor! I ran forward to turn off the tap and went sliding into the cabinet, catching my small toe on the edge of the washing machine and falling backwards into the foam. This did nothing to cushion the blow, my head bouncing off the lino-covered concrete! I got up quickly due to the hot water splashing into my face, and I turned off the hot tap, bending down with one hand wrapped around my toes from the throb and the other on the back of my head.

I cleaned up the foam and must say the kitchen floor came up brilliantly. I opened the back door to help dry it and made a coffee, returning to the living room to relax for a while.

Not long had passed, and someone at the window caused me to jump in fright, a neighbour from down the road.

I put my hearing aid on, realising at this point the television volume was up loud, turning it off I went to the front door and opened it.

The neighbour stood at the door, holding a red card.

"Got a parcel for me mate?" He said.

"No," I said. "Nothing here for anyone."

"You sure?" He asked.

"Yes," I said. "Nothing has been delivered today."

He handed me the card.

"That is number thirty-six," I said. "This is forty-six."

"Oh bloody hell," The man said looking at the card. "This is my fourth attempt today."

"Forth attempt?" I said curiously.

"Yeah," He said. "Came round this morning, no reply, then a couple of times an hour ago but you ignored the door, then just now but I heard the TV."

"Oh sorry about that," I said. "I don't wear hearing aids indoors."

"Why not?" He asked.

"Because I don't," I said.

"Not fair on people that come round is it?" He said. "What if I had an emergency and needed something?"

"Like what?" I asked.

"Ambulance?" He said.

"I don't have any ambulances," I said. "Not got room on the drive for any."

"You know what I mean!" He scoffed, chuckling.

"If I know someone is coming round, then I expect them," I said. "Anyway need to shoot."

"Sure," He said and walked away.

I then returned to finish off the cleaning, including cutting the grass, with no hearing aids on obviously.

An hour into cutting the grass, a parcel was dumped over my gate….. For the neighbour…

119

TINNITUS

I get tinnitus all the time, every day in some annoying way and it is depressing and irritating.

It usually hits me when I am trying to focus or do something chilled.

> "How is your tinnitus?" The audiologist asked me.
> "Really bad," I said. "It's getting to me."
> "Have you tried baths?" She asked. "Swimming also helps."
> "Tried all that," I said.
> "Do you take out your hearing aids or sleep with them in?" She said writing notes.
> "Take them out," I said. "The moulds are way too uncomfortable to wear."
> "Have you tried whale songs?" She said.
> "Yes," I said with a grin. "But can only hold my breath under the water for so long."

She gave me a hearing test, but like most of them, the tinnitus interfered with the results as I struggled to know what was real and what was in my head….. A bit like the voices….

I was on a training course, and I was feeling tired due to the lack of sleep, so tired I was regretting sitting through the training. I had already read the manual due to the fact I struggled to follow what the trainer was talking about, especially with going off-topic with the questions.

One of the delegates, whom I had joined for dinner, decided to sit next to me and I struggled to understand him due to the strong accent.

> "You okay?" One of the delegates asked me.
> "Tired," I said. "Barely slept."
> "Too much booze?" He laughed.
> "No," I said. "Tinnitus."
> "What is that?" He asked curiously."
> "Sounds in my ears," I explained. "More electrical signals."
> "I am confused," He said. "You said you were deaf."
> "I am," I nodded.
> "So how can you hear sounds then?" He asked curiously.

"Hard to explain," I said. "Just google it."

I wasn't in the mood to explain things.

"So are you lying?" He asked. "I bet you can hear."
"I am deaf," I said. "Profoundly."

He covered his mouth and said, "What am I saying?"

"What am I saying," I repeated. "And the only reason I guessed, was because that has been done more times than I can imagine."

He got out his mobile and looked through Google.

"Acupuncture works," He said. "Whale songs apparently." He smiled.
"I tried that," I replied. "But sticking my head in the water and lipreading whales is hard work."
"You can lipread whales!?" He scoffed in amazement.
"Sarcasm," I said. "Wasted on you."
"Can you lipread any animals?" He asked.
"What do you think?" I said.
"Well apes are very similar," He said. "Can you lipread them?"
"You do know animals cannot speak," I replied. "So lipreading is pretty much a no-go."
"Oh," He nodded. "Fair enough."

I looked at him unimpressed, but in my head, I was imagining beating him with a baseball bat.

"Everything okay?" The trainer asked.
"We were talking about lipreading animals," The delegate said.
"Well you were," I said.
"How about you concentrate on the course and not on the fact that if David can lipread animals," He said.
"Whales," I said. "Whales and their songs mainly."

It became a funny discussion at lunchtime and woke me up a fair bit.

121

TODDLER!

I was the first bus of the journey home, having stood for the first half of the journey due to it being full. I was happy when I finally got to sit down due to a knee issue that had plagued me for a couple of weeks.

It was dark out and raining hard, I was on my phone watching videos, as well as the two plastic bottles rolling back and forth, irritating everyone.

I felt a slap on the back of the head and turned around to find a young mother holding a toddler, so I smiled and turned around.

Another slap, slightly harder, so I turned around again.

"What?" The girl said. "She is only playing."
"Not everyone likes getting slapped," I said and grinned, listening to her muttering as I turned around.

Another slap caught my ear.

"Could you not let him do that please," I said.
"She is a girl!" She said in annoyance. "Can't you tell?"
"No," I said. "But can you not let her do that and try and discourage it?"
"She is a toddler!" She said. "She is learning."

I shook my head and turned around and the kid slapped me again.

"How would you like it if I sat behind you and slapped you on the head?" I asked her.
"I'd like to see you try," She laughed and moved the toddler onto the other side of her lap. "Got to move you because this nasty man isn't any fun."

I turned around.

"Getting grief from a Madam attitude because she wants her kid to slap strangers on a bus," I muttered, getting a laugh from the old couple opposite me."

My implant processor was pulled off my head, and that annoyed me, So I turned around.

"What?" She looked at me.
"Your kid has just ripped my hearing aid off my head," I said. "Could I have it back?"
"Drop that," She said to the kid. "It's dirty!" She slapped the kid's hand until she dropped it on the floor and then kicked it into the middle of the aisle.
"Ten grand," I said. "Kids these days have no respect for other people or their property."
"You should have taken it off then," She said. "That way my kid wouldn't have touched it."
"Most people teach their kids manners and right from wrong," I said. "Obviously your mother failed at the same thing."
"You cannot talk to me like that," She said.
"You are the one acting like a complete chav in front of everyone," I said looking around. "Is anyone coming to your aid?" I looked around. "Stop abusing people on the bus just because you think you are owed something."

I turned round and ignored her, yapping and ranting in my ear and after a few minutes, I turned around, smiling at her as I removed it and put it into my pocket.

When the bus came to a stop several minutes later, she struggled with her buggy and looked around.

"Anyone gonna help me or what?" She demanded.
"What?" I said. "Cannot hear you," I pointed to my ears.

As she left, I got a couple of finger signs as she stropped off.

TRAIN ANNOUNCEMENTS

Not a fan of public transportation, but there are times when I have no choice but to use it. I was going into London for a date, nervous as hell but we had spoken for a while and decided just to meet for a coffee and see how the day goes and where it takes us.

I got onto the train to London Victoria, checking the platform screens when the train screen was out of use.

I sat down, texted the girl I was due to meet in London and then randomly looked through videos.

An announcement blared but I had no idea what was said and didn't take any notice.

The train stopped at Bromley South and a woman sat opposite me, smiling.

"Does this go to Victoria?" She asked me.
"Yes," I said.
"Thanks," she replied and then proceeded to have a conversation with someone on the phone.

Several minutes in, the train stopped for some time, long enough for me to wonder what was going on.

"What is happening?" I asked the woman.
"No idea," She said. "Hope it isn't too long."

I got up and had a look around and returned to the seat, to find the woman gone, I then sat down, checking the messages to find my date had messaged me to say she was late.

The train moved and I didn't take much notice, glad it was on the way.

Several minutes passed and the train pulled up at Bromley South and I then thought I was losing it. I saw an attendant and called him over.

"Excuse me," I said. "I am sure we stopped here earlier?"

"Yes," The man said. "There are problems with the line, so the train has reversed its journey," He smiled. "Did you not hear the announcement?"

"No," I replied. "Deaf," I pointed to my implant. "How do I get to London?"

"They are putting up a replacement bus service," He said. "There will be delays."

"Crap," I mumbled.

"Shame the display isn't working," I pointed. "That would be a great help to someone who is deaf."

"Did you not request assistance?" The man asked.

"I cannot request assistance every time I go out," I said. "Would have thought a simple display would be working."

"It's out of action," He said. "Apologies for that. Can I help with anything?"

"No," I said. "I'll get the bus into London."

I got off the train and made my way to the bus stop, looking at my mobile to find a couple of messages.

The date had been cancelled due to issues getting to London and wanted to meet another day. I was unable to get a train back to Longfield, so I got a couple of buses, stopping at Bluewater shopping centre, getting dinner and then a movie. Managed to meet up with a friend, so the day wasn't lost, however, the ridiculously long journey home was.

TRAIN TOILETS

I never use train toilets, they are usually in such a bad state, that it isn't worth the risk. However, on this day, I had no choice.

I had been to London to meet a friend and must have eaten something bad, because once I got on the train, my stomach started rumbling, and cramping. I was a good hour or so from home and knew for a fact, I was either going to throw up or lose control of my bowels.

I sat in the corner of the train, focusing and breathing through it, sweating heavily.

"Are you drunk?" A woman said looking at me from the seat across from me.
"No," I replied. "Something I ate."
"I saw you stumble," She said. "You are drunk."
"I have balance issues," I said. "Due to being deaf, two drinks is hardly going to make me drunk."
"If you say so," She rolled her eyes. "You look drunk."
"Well you look stoned," I said. "Not making an issue of it am I?"

She got up and stormed off, giving me a disapproving look as she went into the next carriage.

In the end, I gave up and headed for the toilet, one of the disabled ones with a revolving door.

I was in there for a while, probably fifteen minutes, fighting the urge to throw up and then I had no choice, it wasn't waiting.

Five minutes later, after feeling a little better and still sitting on the toilet, the door opened and a member of staff and two members of the public stood there, suddenly turning away.

"What the hell?!" I yelped as the door closed.

Feeling better, I then washed my hands and opened the door, finding the member of staff standing there looking rather embarrassed.

"What was that about?" I asked.

126

"We thought there was an emergency," He said.

"There was," I replied. "Trust me."

"We called and knocked, but got no response from you," he said.

"I am deaf," I said. "Couldn't hear anything over the noise of the train."

"Someone saw you walk in and said you looked very unwell," He said. "And when no one responded, we thought you had collapsed."

"It's fine," I said.

"If you want to make a complaint," He took a pad from his pocket. "I will give you my details."

"It's fine," I replied. "Hardly your fault."

"Are you okay, looking a little pale," He stepped back when my stomach gurgled.

"Something I ate has disagreed with me," I said. "This toilet is disgusting," I groaned. "Are they ever cleaned?"

"They are," He said. "People are pretty disgusting."

"I am going to need a tetanus," I groaned.

"We are approaching Longfield Station," He said. "Where are you getting off?"

"There," I said. "I need fresh air, a cool shower and sleep!"

"Do you want to sit down?" He asked.

"No thanks," I replied.

I got off and walked home, a half-hour walk with the breeze against me and luckily, no further issues. Not until the next day anyhow, that was the last time I ate prawns.

TRAPPED

Several years ago, I was doing some medical equipment servicing for a contractor, helping out at a local trust. This was late in the evening after agreeing on a suitable time to come in when treatments and visits had finished.

I was aware that it was a locked facility for mental health patients, and was told what to expect, however, this was not an issue. Getting into the building with an intercom system proved difficult, especially as I didn't have staff access to this part of the building.

I had pressed the buzzer on the intercom, the camera light blinding me unexpectedly.

"Yes?" A female voice on the end.
"Hi," I said. "I am Dave, I am an engineer and I am working on site this evening."
"Okay," The voice replied and the intercom switched off.

I stood around for a few minutes and the door was not opened, so I tried again.

"Yes?" A male voice this time.
"I am an engineer and need to access the site," I replied. "Spoke to someone earlier but no one has let me in."
"Wait there," The man said.

A few minutes later the door opened, and a male nurse, short and stocky in his sixties looked me up and down.

"Why are you here?" He said. "Visiting times are finished."
"I am an engineer," I replied. "Kathy is expecting me."
"Ah," He nodded. "For the yearly service of our treatment room?"
"Yes," I said, struggling to lip-read him.
"Come in and wait by the counter," He said propping the door open. "I will get Kathy."

I stood by the counter for some time and it was cold in the waiting area, and strangely enough, it was colder than it was outside!

After ten minutes of thinking I had been forgotten about, the hall door opened and Kathy walked out, a tall skinny nurse with a very unhappy expression.

"Are you Dave?" She said.

"Yes," I nodded. "I am here to service four items in your treatment room."

"Okay," She said. "Do you have any sharp objects with you?" She looked at my bag.

"No," I said and opened the bag. "Just a tester, wipes and labels. Also a notepad and pen."

"Please do not give anything to any of the patients," She said. "Also keep hold of your mobile, do not let it out of your sight."

"No problems," I replied. "I saw the email from you."

"I will have to look you in the room," She said. "We have vulnerable patients, and also some violent patients, so it's your safety more than theirs."

"That is fine," I said.

"How long will you need?" She said looking at her watch.

"Half an hour to forty-five minutes," I said. "Won't take long."

She walked me to the treatment room, putting on the lights and pointing out the equipment. There is a workshop running the length of the room with various items on it, a sink and draining board at the centre, under a window with metal bars across them. On one side of the room a treatment couch, old and torn, on the other side various locked cabinets, drug fridges and shelving with equipment.

"I will be back in forty-five minutes to let you out," She said. "If there is an emergency, pull the cord," She pointed to a red cord hanging down by a treatment couch. "The equipment is there," She pointed to the worktop. "Do you need anything?"

"No thanks," I said, placing my bag on the worktop.

"Tea or coffee?" She asked.

"No," I said. I already needed the toilet and didn't want to add to that.

"Good," She smiled. "It's bloody horrible in this place!"

She walked out, locking the door behind her and giving me a thumbs-up before walking off.

I serviced the equipment in half an hour, cleaning it up and then placing it back on the worktop. Realising I had some time, I explored the room, reading posters, looking at other items and walking around.

129

"I really need the loo," I thought to myself, regretting the bottle of water I had finished in the car before coming in.

Walking to the door and looking through the window, I looked up the dark corridor to see if I could get someone's attention.

"Hello?" I knocked a couple of times. "Can someone let me out?"

No signs of life, I looked around the room before looking out the door again.

I then got the fright of my life when a young woman appeared at the door, wearing black jogging bottoms and a white t-shirt with tea or coffee stains down the front, her lips cracked and blistered, her long frizzy hair, messy and hanging over her face.

"Hi," I said.

She looked back at me, grinning and looking around, practically rolling her eyes.

"Can you get a nurse for me?" I asked.

She shook her head to say no and laughed.

"Please," I said. "I need a wee."

She knocked on the glass, waved at me and then walked away.

"Shit," I thought. I really needed the toilet, and the bloody dripping tap was not helping. I even thought of using the sink but knowing my luck, someone would walk in.

I waited for another fifteen minutes and was starting to suffer, my bladder felt as if it was going to pop. I returned to the door again, looking for someone only to see the same woman walking up and down, knocking on random doors and walls.

I looked at the cord, tempted to pull it, but it wasn't an emergency and I didn't want to cause that kind of mess, but at the same time, losing control of my bladder would be considered a mess.

I noticed a telephone and decided to try my luck and call reception, hoping the person would be clearly spoken.

I dialled zero and put the phone on speaker, listening as it rang out.

"Yes," A man on the end said.

"Hi," I replied. "Firstly, I am deaf so may struggle. I am an engineer on the ward, I think I have been forgotten about and I am locked in the treatment room."

"Are you a patient?" The man asked.

"No," I replied. "I am a contractor."

"Do you have a contact?" He asked.

I had forgotten the name of the nurse, my mind completely blank.

"I cannot remember her name," I said. "I also need the toilet and not sure how much I can hold on," I said looking at the tap. "Plus there is a leaking tap in here, torturing the crap out of me."

"Stay there," He said and hung up.

I was waiting a few minutes when someone knocked on the treatment room door.

"Who are you?" The male nurse said. "Why are you in there?"

"I am an engineer," I replied. "Doing some servicing on site."

"Any identification?" He asked.

"No," I said.

"I am going to get security," He replied.

"Kathy," I remembered. "Kathy knows I am working here."

"Right," The nurse said and walked away.

"Give me a break!" I moaned, close to bursting.

A few minutes later, Kathy showed up and unlocked the door looking very distressed.

131

"I am so sorry," She said. "I got distracted with a patient and completely forgot you were here!"

"It's fine," I said. "Is there a loo?"

"Not here no," She said. "Ours are for staff only."

"Great," I said.

"Did you do everything?" she asked.

"Yes," I replied. "All done, I need to go now."

As I walked out of the door, the patient from earlier came running up to me and giving me a bear hug, practically hanging off me.

I managed to find some toilets in the main reception and felt a lot better once I left. I have never been back, but who knows? If I ever lose the plot, maybe they will have a room put by for me.

RADIO LOOP STAR

Back in school and eventually at college, I had a Radio microphone and receiver. This was used in a classroom setting where I wore the radio receiver with a loop, and the teacher would wear a microphone.

I never particularly liked using it, due to it being too loud, and too much interference and every time there was a loud noise, I would launch in the air with fright.

When I was at mainstream school, it was an afternoon mock exam. I had missed the questions, despite the teacher reading them out twice, however with his thick beard and accent, I struggled to understand him.

"Excuse me, sir," I said raising my hand.
"Be quiet during the test," He said.
"But I didn't hear the question," I said. "Could you repeat it?"
"No," He snapped. "When I say not to speak, I expect you to listen!"

That shut me up...

I sat there feeling lost and nervous, and to be honest, it was the norm for me.

"I am going to the toilet," He said. "Carry on and if there is any messing around, detention will be given out to everyone."

The teacher then left the room, completely oblivious that he had forgotten the radio microphone.

From there I could hear him walking down the corridor to the toilet at the end, mumbling and whistling. The sound of the door closing, the toilet stall door closing and the sound of the toilet seat slamming down.

"Oh dear," I said quietly, several students shushing me and giving me evil looks. One guy sitting on my side, well known for bulling people but had rarely bothered me, leaned over, and punched me in the arm, holding up his finger in warning.

The teacher continued to mumble, grunt as well as the occasional fart and water splash.

The toilet flushed and he fumbled around with his belt.

"Not finished," He said and then proceeded to urinate, the sound of the stream hitting the water echoing in my ears, so I turned down the volume.

A few minutes later, he returned to the room and checked his watch before sitting down.

"Pens down!" He said loudly and then looked at me. "What was it you wanted?"
"I didn't hear the question," I said.
"Then why didn't you ask me to repeat it?!" He bellowed.
"I tried," I said. "But you had a go at me."
"Don't speak to me with that attitude," He said. "I will not have any of your attitude in here!"

He tapped the microphone, causing me to jump.

"Can you hear this?!" He bellowed.
"Yes," I replied. "Don't do that."
"Why couldn't you hear the question?" He asked.
"Because I couldn't understand," I said.
"Does this work?" He fiddled with the microphone.
"Yes," I replied. "I heard you go to the toilet, pee and fart."

The room erupted in laughter.

"How dare you!" He said. "Come here!"

I got up and walked over to the table, nervously.

"Hold out your hand!" He demanded.

I held out my hand, palm down.

"Turn it," He said. "Palm upwards."

I turned my hand.

"This is what happens to children that mess around in my classroom!" He said, pulling a ruler from the draw and without warning, brought it down on my hand.

The pain made my eyes water and I didn't show any emotion, keeping it locked up inside and screaming silently.

"Did that hurt?" He asked me.

For some stupid reason, I said no.

He brought the ruler down again, the snapping crack echoing around the room. I hissed in pain, putting my hand under my arm.

"Now go to the headmaster!" He demanded. "Take this rubbish with you!" He pulled off the receiver, shoving it into my hand. "Get out of my classroom!"

I walked out, in tears.

I got to the headmaster's office, standing outside.

The headmaster, a tall and serious-looking man who was also the local scout leader, was someone I had an unfortunate encounter with again when joining the scouts. He told me to come into the room.

"Well it appears you have been playing up," He said. "What do you have to say for yourself?"

I explained what had happened, however he seemed to have no sympathy for me.

"Give me that!" He held his hand out.

I handed him the radio microphone and he dropped it onto the table.

135

"I will not have this behaviour in school," He said. "Stand against the table and turn around."
"Why?" I asked nervously.
"Do NOT question me!" He snapped. "Do what you are told!"

I flinched, turned around and stood against the table.

He then started to speak, but I couldn't see him to be able to lip-read him, so I turned around.

"What did I tell you!" He growled, grabbing me by the shoulder and aggressively turning me around.

Panicking inside as I tried to listen, my nervousness was met with a sharp searing pain on my backside, followed by another four, one catching me on the lower back causing me to jolt and my glasses to fall off. Each time he hit me, the amplified slap echoed in my ears through the loop system.

I bit my tongue, my eyes watering as I fought back tears.

"Turn around!" He said.

I picked up my glasses and turned around to find him putting his plimsole back on, looking at me in disgust.

"I wish I had a cane," He said. "You need discipline, I don't want to hear any more excuses when you are told to do something, you will do it!"
"Yes sir," I said, my voice breaking.
"Now get back to class," He said. "You have detention every evening for an extra hour and I will send a letter to your parents!"

I started to walk towards the door.

"Hey!" He called out. "Don't forget that!" He pointed to the radio microphone. "Maybe you need to turn it up so you can hear what the teachers are saying, and maybe concentrate!"

I limped back to the classroom, my eyes teary and my throat raw.

The teacher showed concern when I sat down in pain, asking me if I were okay, but I nodded and got on with my work.

COLLEGE FUN

I had an updated radio loop at college, given to me by the local audiology support, I didn't want it as I found it no help, especially in group settings, but they said to keep it in case.

On one chilled study day, a group of us were bored and a friend of mine asked if I had it, seeing as we had fun with it at one point.

"Let's play a game," He said. "We could do with a laugh!"
"What?" I said. "What do you have in mind?"
"You will see," He said, taking the radio kit from my bag.

I put on the loop and he had the microphone.

"Go out into the field," He said pointing to the football post in the field in front of the theatre.

I walked out into the field, listening as the interference grew the further away I got.

"Stop!" His voice echoed in my ears.

I stopped.

"Turn around," He said.

I didn't catch it so I listened again.

"Turn, around!" he said again.

I turned around and faced him, along with a few others.

"Jump up and down!" He said.

I jumped up and down, hearing them laughing.

"Walk backwards and dance!" He said.

I walked backwards and danced, making a complete fool of myself, noticing more people watching the show.

"Take off your t-shirt," He said.

I held up my arms in confusion.

"Take off your t-shirt!" He said again.

I didn't have a clue, so I took off my shoe, causing him to burst into fits of laughter.

It then started to rain and the interference was louder and annoying. Turning off the microphone, I ran back to the group.

"That was hysterical!" One of the girls said. "Can I have a go?"
"No!" I said. "It's horrible."
"Have you got the alarm clock?" My friend asked.
"No," I said curiously. "Why?"
"What are you talking about?" The girl said.
"I have a vibrating alarm clock!" I said.
"Oh wow!" She smiled curiously.
"No," I said. "Definitely not!"
"Spoilsport!" She said.

I stayed over at a house a year or so later and had my alarm clock stolen at some point, and I am pretty sure it was one of the girls.....

WASTE OF TIME

I was sat in the reception of an office building in London, watching as various people came and went. The interviews were running late, and I had already been sitting waiting for nearly an hour, bored silly.

"Mr Blackwell?" The receptionist asked. Not sure why she was confirming considering she had already spoken to me a couple of times.

"Yes?" I replied.

"The manager will be down for you shortly," She smiled. "Are you sure you cannot do a telephone interview? It would make his life much easier."

"Not unless you have cured deafness?" I said grinning. "Then I would be more than happy to."

"No," She said seriously. "We haven't," She sighed. "Is there no way you could try?"

"Try to what?" I asked. "Not be deaf?"

She laughed awkwardly and walked away, hurrying when one of the reception telephones started to ring.

"Mental," I thought to myself.

"How deaf are you?" The woman opposite me asked.

"Severe," I replied. "I need hearing aids and to be able to lipread to communicate."

"Oh wow that is amazing," She said. "You do so well."

The receptionist walked over again.

"I have been asked to double check you are unable to use the telephone," She said.

"Same answer to the last ten times I was asked," I replied. "If someone was in a wheelchair, would you keep asking them to climb the stairs?"

The woman opposite me laughed.

"Well no," The receptionist said. "They are in a wheelchair and they cannot walk, so that would be silly."

"But the fact I am deaf and cannot hear on the telephone is too difficult for you to understand?" I said.

"No," She said. "You speak fine, so that is why I am confused."

"No comment," I said. What I was going to say, wouldn't have gone down well. (Well you don't look stupid considering you are.)

She nodded and walked back to the reception, picking up the telephone and speaking to someone, looking at me at the same time.

"Not very good is it?" The woman said to me. "Would you really want to work for them?"

"No," I replied. "But it seems to be a common issue everywhere."

"Really?" She said in surprise. "What is the interview for?"

"IT support," I said.

"Best of luck," The woman said.

Several minutes passed and a man in a three-piece suit came out from a room next to reception, yelling across for my attention. I got up and walked over to him.

"David?" He said. "Can you hear me?"

"Yes," I replied.

"So how come you couldn't do the interview over the telephone?" He asked.

"I need to lip-read," I replied.

"What is that?" He asked curiously.

"Reading lips," I said. "It's how I communicate."

"Odd," He said. "Not heard of that before."

"Lip patterns," I replied. "Along with sound."

"Learn something new every day," He nodded. "Come though."

I followed him into the room, and there was a desk at the centre with a laptop and various papers scattered all over the desk, along with three cups of coffee, half untouched.

"Drink?" He asked.

"No," I said. "I have a doctor's appointment soon," I looked at my watch. "Wasn't expecting things to run late."

"I had to sort out something for my wife," He said. "It's her birthday, so busy weekend."

I sat down.

"Before we start," He said. "How deaf are you?"

"Severe," I replied. "I rely on lipreading and hearing aids."

"Wow that is amazing," He said. "Never met a deaf person before so wasn't sure how to react."

"Nothing special," I smiled.

"How did you go deaf?" He asked.

"Unknown," I said.

"Anyone else deaf?" He said.

"No offence," I said. "But I would rather just do the interview."

"Sorry, but the job has been filled," He said sitting down. "That is why I wanted to speak to you on the telephone."

"If the job was filled, why was I invited to an interview?" I said in annoyance.

"It was filled this morning," He chuckled. "A friend of mine."

"Nothing to do with the fact I am deaf?" I said.

"No," He shook his head. "But you wouldn't be suitable."

"Why not?" I asked.

"Because you are deaf," He said bluntly. "You need to be able to hear on the phone."

"That wasn't in the job description," I said.

"Didn't need to be," He said. "We were not expecting a deaf person to apply."

I stood up.

"Might be an idea to put that on your job description," I said. "Disabled people need not apply."

"That is a bit much," he laughed.

"You have wasted my day," I said. "Left me waiting nearly an hour because you were faffing around with private work."

"I am a manager," He said. "That is what I do."

"They pay you to do personal things at work?" I asked.

"No," He laughed nervously.

"I will be complaining to the job centre," I said. "And also complaining to this company about the treatment I have received today."

"It isn't personal," he said.

"Well you offered the role to your friend before you completed the interviews," I said. "I am pretty sure that will raise some concerns."

"How about I see if there are other jobs going," he said. "How about sales?"

"How about no?" I said, walking to the door. "People like you are the reason discrimination thrives."

I walked out of the room and into reception where the woman I had spoken to earlier was at the desk.

"How did it go?" She asked me in front of several people.

"He offered the job to one of his mates," I said. "And that my hearing issue is a problem for them."

"You are joking!" She scoffed.

"Unfortunately not," I replied. "This kind of thing is quite common due to idiots that have issues with disabilities."

I walked out angry and frustrated, complaining to both the company and the job centre.

Nothing was looked into or done about it but saying that the job centres were even worse when it came to deaf awareness.

The number of times I explained I was deaf, and they kept putting me forward to jobs requiring telephone work.

Not much has changed in the last twenty years, unfortunately.

HEARING AID THEIF

When I was at secondary school not long after starting, I was nervous and didn't have any friends. A friend decided he no longer wanted to be friends with me, so it was back to square one and being deaf made it harder.

At lunchtime, I would hide in the fields, making up stories in my head just to pass the time.

It was one of those days when I knew things would suck. A girl came over to me asking if I wanted to be friends only for her to retract it and laugh at me, her friends joining in.

I found a quiet spot at the bottom of the field, hiding in a gap in the trees where no one could see me, or so I thought.

I was halfway through my cheese rolls when a couple of older boys walked in with a girl.

"What are you doing in our smoking spot?" One of the boys said.
"Sorry," I said. "I will leave."
"Oh let him stay," The girl said.

The boys lit up cigarettes, offering one to the girl who refused.

"You want one?" He asked me.
"No," I said.
"Why not?" He asked.
"I don't want one," I said, finishing my roll and putting the other back in the bag.
"What's that?" He pointed to my hearing aid.
"Hearing aid," I said.
"Why?" He said. "You a retard or something?"
"No," I said nervously. "I am deaf."
"Aww!" The girl said.

One of the boys leaned forward, grabbing the hearing aid off my ear.

"Hey come on!" I said nervously. "I need that."

He then grabbed the other one, knocking off my glasses which I quickly picked up and put into my bag.

"Give them back please," I begged.

The boy then left, running out into the field, followed by the other boy and girl, laughing all the way out of the bushes.

Grabbing my bag, I ran out and followed them across the field towards the bridge.

When I finally caught up with them, the other boy came at me and kicked my legs from under me. They all laughed as I fell heavily to the floor, lying in a heap winded.

They then left me there, running off.

I eventually got up and went to the audiology, dreading it as the audiologist hated me.

"What happened?" She asked. "Sit down," She pointed to a chair.

I explained what had happened, and she sighed heavily, shaking her head.

"This seems to happen to you a lot," She said. "Do you go out looking for trouble?"
"No," I said tearfully.
"Where did you lose them?" She demanded.
"I didn't," I said. "An older boy stole them."
"Rubbish," She said. "Why would someone steal your hearing aids?"
"I don't know," I said.

She leaned over to check my ears, smelling my blazer.

"Have you been smoking!" She snapped.
"No," I said. "The boys were smoking."

144

There was a knock at the door and the audiologist sat back.

"Wait there," She said and got up.

A few minutes passed, and she came back, holding my hearing aids.

"Well a student just returned these," She said. "They found them in the bushes at the bottom of the field where people smoke," She sighed in frustration. "Why were you there?"

"I was there for lunch," I said. "I thought I would be safe there,"

"Safe from what?" she said. "Safe to smoke?"

"I don't smoke!" I said in annoyance.

"Well the student said he saw you smoking," She said. "I will have to report this to the headmaster."

I had given up at this point. It didn't matter what I did or said, I knew it wouldn't go my way.

I was sent over to the headmaster's office and was called in immediately.

"So," He said. "David," He sat back in his chair. "What do you have to say for yourself?"

"Nothing," I said.

"You were smoking," He sighed. "I am very disappointed."

"I was not smoking, I was there for lunch," I argued.

"Why were you there?" He asked.

At this point, I broke down and cried.

"Come on stop that," He said. "Tell me why you hide?"

"Because I get bullied," I said. "It doesn't matter what I do, I get bullied!"

"Three students saw you smoking," He said. "And that you left your hearing aids there."

"Not true," Is said.

"You also swore at them when they spoke to you and tried to give you your hearing aids back," He said. "That wasn't very nice."

"They are lying," I said. "I was there having my lunch and they took my hearing aids, they were the ones smoking."

"Why would they lie?" He said. "Why are you making things up?"

145

"I am not making things up," I said through tears.

"An hour detention after school," He said. "Report to the afterschool room."

"But sir!" I complained. "I didn't do anything!"

"Do you want another hour?" He warned me.

I went to detention as ordered, no matter what I said or did, I wasn't listened to.

And the issue didn't end there.

I was due to help out at the school farm after school, people would volunteer for an hour or so to help with cleaning, feeding and so on. I asked someone to let the science teacher know, that I would not be able to join.

When I got to the room, I was the only person there. The teacher, reading a book asked me for my form from the headmaster. They had three colours for 'lines', blue, yellow and green, depending on the year.

"Green," She snapped.

"Green what?" I asked.

I had never done this before, so it was alien to me.

"Green lines!" She said. "At the back, two sheets to be done in an hour."

That was two hundred lines with the sentence "I must no smoke and lie at school".

After half an hour, I was three-quarters of the way through the lines when the teacher came up to me.

"How are you doing?" she asked.

I showed her the forms.

"Good," She said. "I am going to the toilet, carry on."

She left the room and I continued to write, my hand aching so badly.

146

The door opened, and the science teacher looked in, red in the face.

"What are you doing?" He said looking at his watch. "You are supposed to be at the farm."
"I got detention," I said. "I did tell someone to let you know."
"Why have you got detention?" He said looking at the sheets. "Smoking and lying?!" He bellowed and slammed his hand down on the table. "I expected better from you David!"

His reaction shook me up.

"Why?" He demanded. "Why are you smoking and lying?"
"I didn't," I said. "Someone took my hearing aids and said I was smoking."
"Just get on with it," He said. "Very disappointed in you!" He slammed his hand on the table again before walking out, closing the door behind him.

The teacher walked in several minutes later.

"Finished?" She asked.

I nodded.

"You still have twenty minutes, so I suggest you do some more," She said.

Not a great day for me, but many more were to follow.

DEAF EXCUSES

I used to work for a mortgage company, it was my second job after working for the hotel and was a little more interesting and paid much better.

I joined a team that would set mortgages up, doing a shift from two in the afternoon to nine in the evening. I didn't mind the hours and it was much quieter after four, giving us time to do what we needed without any interruptions.

A new manager joined, and she was always on someone's case and I was not immune. On her second day, she called me into her office.

"Sit down please," She said pointing to a chair and looking at a file with my name on it.

I smiled and sat down, a notebook and pen in my hand.

"It is just a review," she said. "I am new so I am speaking to everyone."
"Okay," I said.
"How long have you been here?" She asked.
"Six months or so," I said.
"And what do you do?" She said.
"I set up mortgages on the system and deal with enquiries," I said. "Also working with the scoring team."
"Good," She said. "Do you enjoy it?"
"It's okay," I said. "Keeps me busy."
"Okay," She nodded. "I have had a couple of complaints about your role."
"How come?" I asked. "What complaints?"
"That you do not pull your weight," She said.
"How do you mean?" I asked curiously.

I was in that mindset where rather than put up with stress or messing around, I would have walked and found a job elsewhere.

"Two people have complained that you are avoiding certain jobs and leaving them to other people," She said. "Therefore creating more work for others."

"Could you give me details please?" I asked.

This woman never looked up from the file once, her eyes scanning through it.

"We are a call centre," She said. "And part of that requires people to pick up a telephone when it rings and assist the person on the end," She sighed and looked up. "We cannot have team members ignoring this."

"Have you read my file correctly?" I said.

"I have amazing attention to detail," She said. "Nothing escapes me."

"How about the part where it states I am deaf?" I said.

She froze, looked down at the paperwork and then back up at me.

"Deaf?" She said. "How did you get a job in a call centre?"

"They wanted to offer me a role," I said. "So the job was changed, so I can then do what is required uninterrupted and help out others where needed," I explained. "I also file."

"That wasn't explained to me," She said.

"It's in my file," I said. "I know that because I was asked to read through it and confirm it."

"Well I have to look into these things," She said. "When people complain, I have to action it."

"I get it," I said. "There will always be people with vendettas."

"How deaf are you?" She asked. "Can you hear on the phone at all?"

"I can hear," I said. "But not well enough to follow a conversation due to relying on lip-reading."

She nodded, looking through the file.

"So can you confirm that you do not use your hearing loss as a reason to get out of work?" She said.

"Are you asking me if I use my hearing disability to get out of work?" I scoffed.

"I have to ask," She said.

"No I don't," I said. "If I could hear on the telephone, trust me, I would pick up the phone that rings constantly and irritates me because someone else would ignore it."

I was fuming.

149

"I would tell those two girls that sit opposite me to answer the phone themselves instead of disappearing to talk to their boyfriends," I said. "Or the constant toilet breaks."

"What makes you think they complained?" She asked.

"Because they complained about the same thing to the last manager," I said. "We had a similar discussion and I said if it happened again, I would take action."

"Action for what?" She asked.

"Discrimination for a start," I said. "You said your attention to detail was good, yet you miss the bit in bold about me being deaf and not able to hear on the phone. This was also agreed when I was given a contract."

"No need to get upset," She said.

"I am not upset," I said. "Just annoyed that despite doing my job, I still have to humour those that don't."

"I will speak to them and assure them it doesn't happen again," She said.

Someone knocked on the door and it opened slowly, revealing one of the men I worked with.

"Hi Dave," He said. "Just to let you know that old couple asked for you."

"Oh no!" I moaned. "Not them again."

We had an elderly couple that had a few properties, and when they came to make payments, it was always in cash. One time I had to count nearly four hundred pounds in coins!

The manager looked at me and smiled.

"Could you ask the two girls to go down and assist," she said. "Dave and I have an important meeting."

Karma hit the two girls who complained about me, and they had to spend a couple of hours counting cash. They were also warned (again) about complaining and told the reasons why.

The manager took me for lunch that day, and we got on well following that.

150

YOU NEED TO HEAR THIS

I was on a course for medical equipment and all was going well until the trainer decided to put me on the spot.

"Can you hear that?" He asked.

There were several people on the course, and despite telling him I was deaf, I am not sure he had listened.

"Here what?" I asked.

He laughed.

"What is the sound?" I asked.
"Don't worry about it," He said and sighed.
"No," I said. "You asked a question so I am following up on it," I breathed out heavily. "What is the sound."
"If you cannot hear it then there is no point," He dismissed me.
"Well of course not," I said. "I am deaf and you are at the end of the table where there are several people around it."
"It doesn't matter," He said.
"I would like to know considering you asked me a question," I said. "What was the sound?"

He groaned.

"Not an unfair question," one of the students said. "Shall I?"
"No," The tutor said. "I will tell him, come here," He called me over.

I got up and walked over to the tutor, looking down at the equipment that was open and plugged into the mains.

"So humour me," I said. "What is making the sound."
"The motor," He said.

151

"Okay," I said.

"It should be humming," He said. "If you hear clicking, then it is faulty."

I bent down, putting my hearing aid closer.

"Nope," I said. "Cannot hear anything."

"Then you cannot service these," He said. "You cannot be deaf and do this job."

"Wow," I said. "I have managed for years and if I cannot hear something, I have colleagues."

"I just think it's silly," The tutor said. "Some jobs shouldn't be done by certain people."

"Well you shouldn't be a trainer considering you have no people skills," I said. "Your attitude sucks."

"No need to be rude," he said. "I will still sign you off."

"And I will still be complaining," I said. "I have never been insulted so much on a training course."

"It was my opinion," He said. "No need to take it the wrong way."

"I will let the company know your opinion," I said. "Discriminatory."

"It was not discrimination," He said.

"You cannot be deaf and do this job," I said. "Pretty clear if you ask me."

Some of the other students agreed.

"Was below the belt," One of the students said. "Besides, as you said, the motor rarely goes wrong."

"I'll take it up with our rep," I said. "No other company has made any issues regarding my hearing disability or told me I cannot do the job like it's the sixties."

"You are blowing this out of proportion," He said, holding up his hands.

"Guess you refuse to train women?" I said.

There were no women on the course.

"Look," He said. "I apologise for my stupid comment, it was ignorant of me."

The rest of the training went well, and he was as nice as a pie.

I also got another apology at the end of the day. It annoyed me, considering something so small was a major issue for the trainer.

MORE BATTERY WOES

I was at the airport as part of my month-long trip to America, and already I knew it was going to be an awkward day. Met by long queues, and a very noisy environment at the security point at Heathrow Airport, I was rummaging through my bag trying to find my spare battery as I had forgotten to charge the one in my implant overnight, and it was beeping, indicating low.

"Bloody annoying," I muttered, stopping when I nearly walked into the couple in front of me. The woman turned around and looked at me. "I was talking to myself," I said smiling. "Lost something."

The woman nodded and forced a smile, pulling her partner closer as they approached the conveyor belt. Her flight pillow was half blown up and barely clinging to her neck.

My implant beeped and that was the final one before I lost all sound within ten minutes or so.

I noticed a security guard standing by the side and asked her to come over to me.

"Hi," I said. "Just wanted to let you know that my battery is going to die and I will be completely deaf."
"No problem darling," She said. "Do you need assistance?"
"No I will be fine, but don't want anyone to think I am ignoring them," I said.
"I will let them know," She said, calling someone on the radio and explaining it, pointing me out.
"Embarrassing," I said softly. "I could do without this."

A security officer called me over to another conveyor belt.

"Do you need help going through security?" He asked.
"No," I said. "Just that I may not be able to hear anyone speaking to me."
"Okay," he said. "I'll keep an eye on things for you."

The woman in front of Ryan turned around, grinning.

"Special treatment?" She said.
"No," I replied. "Why?"

153

"How come you are getting help then?" She asked.

"Not sure it is any of your business," I said.

"Wow," She scoffed and turned around.

"If I were getting special treatment," I said. "I'd be on the other side by now."

I closed my eyes and shook my head in frustration as the implant battery died, that was a short ten minutes.

Placing my bags on the conveyor, I watched people around me to hopefully copy them without any issues. Noticing a green light near the desk, I planned to use that as his queue to exit the tube.

"This is going to be fun," I said watching the woman from in front of me get into a large scanning booth, positioning her legs on the markings and placing her hands on the front, looking up as the scanner whizzed around. Noticing the woman responding to commands from the operator, Ryan knew he was going to struggle.

"You now sir," The woman behind the screen bluntly said, pointing towards the scanner and not looking up from the screen.

I moved closer so I could see her lips.

"Hi," I said. "I am completely deaf so will struggle," I explained.

"Stand in the scanner please sir," She said. "Very straightforward."

"Okay," I said. "Made you aware."

"Just position your feet and hands on the markings and look up," She said and nodded uninterested as I walked over to the scanner, waiting for the doors to open.

"Let the fun begin," I said and stepped into the scanner, putting my feet on the markings, then my hands and then looked up. I watched as the scanner whizzed around, looking for the green light out of the corner of my eye.

I looked at the desk and the woman looked up, annoyed.

"Don't move," She said. "I will do it again," She indicated to me. "Put your hands on the circles and wait."

I put my hands on the circles, looking to see if he could see the green light.

"Come on," I muttered to myself. "I want some breakfast!"

There was no green light, and the door didn't open so I stayed still, just in case. A few seconds later the door opened and the woman appeared in front of the scanner, looking frustrated and put out.

"Why are you not listening?" She demanded.
"What?" I said. I could barely lip-read her.
"I have been giving you commands," She shook her head. "You are holding people up."
"I did tell you that I couldn't hear," I said to her.
"Then focus," She said. "Follow my instructions."
"I would if I could lip-read you," I said. "Focusing doesn't help me when I am completely deaf."

The woman paused, looking at Ryan and then at another security officer who shrugged his shoulders.

"You cannot hear anything?" She asked.
"Nothing," I said.
"Then why didn't you say something?" She asked. "You should have said."
"I did," I said. "But you kept telling me to look up and not move," I argued. "I cannot do both."
"Okay," She said. "You can go," She waved me away rudely.
"Thanks," I said, walking over to the end of the conveyor to collect my bags, noticing the camera bag wasn't there. "Do you know where the camera bag is?" I asked a woman at the end of the conveyor, collecting the trays.

Turns out my bag was being held for inspection as I accidentally left a small screwdriver kit in the side, the security guard was very understanding and let me sort out my implant before we agreed to dispose of the screwdriver set, something easily replaced when I got to the states.

LIFE CHANGING

When I first started at the hospital as a volunteer, I regularly saw this girl who also worked there and we always briefly chatted. I liked her quite a bit, however being the way I am, I never did anything about it.

Fast forward many years later, I was walking through the hospital and we saw each other again, this was nearly eighteen years later.

"Hey," She said. "Remember me?" She asked.
"Of course," I said. "How are you?"
"Great," She smiled. "Still here I see!"
"Stuck here!" I laughed. "How is life treating you?"
"Married with kids," She laughed. "Working in my local pharmacy."
"Oh cool," I said. "How many kids?"
"Two," She scoffed. "Too many! Are you still volunteering?"
"No," I said. "Working for medical engineering now."
"Big change then," She said. "You free at the moment, fancy a coffee?"

We decided to go and grab a coffee, she was visiting a relative and still had some time before going.

"So what about you?" She asked. "Married? Kids?"
"No," I said. "Never had the luck."
"Why?" She asked curiously.
"No Idea," I said. "Don't seem to have any interest from the ladies."
"Not true," She said. "I was interested."

My heart went nuts at this point.

"What?" I said in disbelief. "When?"
"When I worked here," She said. "We used to see each other all the time, and I put it down to you stalking me!" She laughed out loud. "I thought, I cannot wait for him to ask, so I decided to make a move one day and you walked away from me," She said.
"I walked away from you?" I said. "I don't remember that."

156

"You said hello and we crossed each other, so I turned around and called you a couple of times, but you walked away," She said. "Guessed you were not interested."

"Hold on," I said. "You do know I am deaf?"

"No," She said. "Are you?"

"Don't tell me you didn't know?" I said. "I was trying to build up the courage to ask you out for months," I groaned. "I was pretty upset when I found out you left!"

"Oh no!" She said. "I just thought you weren't interested!"

"Oh bloody hell!" I said. "I should have asked you out!"

We laughed about it and agreed that everything happens for a reason.

My hearing disability does a good job of getting in the way of potential relationships!

Printed in Great Britain
by Amazon